MW00335239

"This is a fascinating book that shows analysis that has been devoted to the s deficits and early trauma. In particular, ᴠ ideas is discussed, comparing them critically and revealing how primitive aspects are edited in the intersubjective analytical field. A useful book not only for the psychoanalyst but also for other professionals dealing with mental health."

Roosevelt Cassorla, Training Analyst of the Psychoanalytic Society of São Paulo, Brazil. Sigourney Award 2017. Author of *The Psychoanalyst, the Theater of Dreams and the Clinic of Enactment* (Routledge).

"We must include Nemirovsky amongst the most necessary of thinkers today, ones who open up new paths for post-Freudian Psychoanalysis, following the stream established by Ferenczi. A century later, contemporary psychoanalists neither work with the same patients nor in the same way of working and listening as before. New paradigms have appeared and they oblige the analyst to create a dialogue between diverse theories. The dialogue proposed by Nemirovsky between Winnicott and Kohut concerning the basis of narcissism and the origins of our subjectivity results in creative and enriching thought which presents us with 'new' ways in which to consider our complex clinical work."

Martina Burdet, IPA Full Member and Training Analyst at the Madrid Psychoanalytical Association (Spain) and Member of the SPP (Société Psychanalytique de Paris). General Secretary of the European Psychoanalytical Federation (EPF).

"This book is a fundamental contribution which reflects contemporary clinical practice. It is a lucid exercise of rereading classic authors in the light of the problems that we currently face in our everyday work.

The author constructs a dialogue between D. Winnicott and H. Kohut that provides us with a rich knowledge of the ideas of these two great pioneers of Psychoanalysis, and goes further as it opens up paths for new developments and thus constitutes an excellent example of how Psychoanalysis can grow looking to the future."

Virginia Ungar, MD, IPA President.

Winnicott and Kohut on Intersubjectivity and Complex Disorders

Given the complexity of scientific developments inside and outside the psychoanalytic field, traditional definitions of basic psychoanalytic notions are no longer sufficiently comprehensive. We need conceptualizations that encompass new clinical phenomena observed in present-day patients and that take into account contributions inside, outside, and on the boundaries of our practice.

This book discusses theoretical concepts which explain current clinical expressions that are as ineffable as they are commonplace. Our patients resort to these expressions when they feel distressed by their perception of themselves as unreal, empty, fragile, non-existent, non-desiring, doubtful about their identity, beset by feelings of futility and apathy, and emotionally numb. The book aims at contrasting the ideas of Winnicott and Kohut, which are connected with a clinical practice that sees each patient as unique and are moreover in direct contact with empirical facts, and applies them to the benefit of complex patients. These ideas facilitate the expansion of paths in both the theory and the practice of our profession.

Uniquely contrasting the works of two seminal thinkers with a Latin American perspective, *Winnicott and Kohut on Intersubjectivity and Complex Disorders* will be invaluable to clinicians and psychoanalysts.

Carlos Nemirovsky, MD, graduated from the Universidad de Buenos Aires in 1969. He is a full member of the Psychoanalytical Association of Buenos Aires and IPA, a training analyst and Professor, Master of Psychoanalysis with the Psychoanalysis Institute of Mental Health, member of IARPP, and President of the Psychoanalytical Association of Buenos Aires from January, 2019.

Winnicott and Kohut on Intersubjectivity and Complex Disorders

New Perspectives for Psychoanalysis, Psychotherapy and Psychiatry

Carlos Nemirovsky

TRANSLATED BY JUDITH FILC
LANGUAGE CONSULTANT EMMET BOLAND

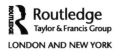

LONDON AND NEW YORK

First published 2021
by Routledge
2 Park Square, Milton Park, Abingdon, Oxon OX14 4RN

and by Routledge
52 Vanderbilt Avenue, New York, NY 10017

Routledge is an imprint of the Taylor & Francis Group, an informa business

© 2021 Carlos Nemirovsky

The right of Carlos Nemirovsky to be identified as author of this
work has been asserted by him in accordance with sections 77 and
78 of the Copyright, Designs and Patents Act 1988.

All rights reserved. No part of this book may be reprinted or
reproduced or utilised in any form or by any electronic, mechanical,
or other means, now known or hereafter invented, including
photocopying and recording, or in any information storage or
retrieval system, without permission in writing from the publishers.

Trademark notice: Product or corporate names may be trademarks
or registered trademarks, and are used only for identification and
explanation without intent to infringe.

British Library Cataloguing-in-Publication Data
A catalogue record for this book is available from the British Library

Library of Congress Cataloging-in-Publication Data
Names: Nemirovsky, Carlos, 1945- author.
Title: Winnicott and Kohut on intersubjectivity and complex
disorders: new perspectives for psychoanalysis, psychotherapy and
psychiatry / Carlos Nemirovsky.
Description: Abingdon, Oxon; New York, NY: Routledge, 2021. |
Includes bibliographical references and index. |
Identifiers: LCCN 2020012624 (print) | LCCN 2020012625 (ebook) |
ISBN 9780367483623 (hardback) | ISBN 9780367483647 (paperback) |
ISBN 9781003039501 (ebook)
Subjects: MESH: Winnicott, D. W. (Donald Woods), 1896–1971. |
Kohut, Heinz. | Psychoanalytic Theory | Interpersonal Relations |
Mental Disorders—therapy | Psychoanalytic Therapy—methods
Classification: LCC RC454 (print) | LCC RC454 (ebook) | NLM WM 460.2 |
DDC 616.89—dc23
LC record available at https://lccn.loc.gov/2020012624
LC ebook record available at https://lccn.loc.gov/2020012625

ISBN: 978-0-367-48362-3 (hbk)
ISBN: 978-0-367-48364-7 (pbk)
ISBN: 978-1-003-03950-1 (ebk)

Typeset in Times New Roman
by codeMantra

To María Alejandra

Contents

Prologue

Valentín Barenblit[1]

Writing the prologue for a book certainly involves a transcendental action in which the most relevant aspects of personal, professional, and ethical commitments converge. On this occasion, the generosity of the author, who has honoured me by asking me to play this role, belies a fact that should be revealed to the readers: I am not a qualified expert in the work of Donald Woods Winnicott or Heinz Kohut, which Carlos Nemirovsky discusses with both excellence and theoretical and clinical rigour. However, I feel I can legitimately provide a brief introduction for several reasons, of which I will mention some. In my view, these justify my having the pleasure of endorsing this book with my thoughts and opinions.

First, I would like to point out the significance of an intellectual and emotional bond that has lasted several decades and defied time and distance. I was forced to go into exile almost 30 years ago and have lived in Barcelona ever since. Yet, as has been the case with my relationship with other colleagues and friends, my connection with Carlos Nemirovsky has endured both intellectually and emotionally. This relationship harks back to our work in, and professional and personal commitment to, the Psychopathology and Neurology Ward of the Aráoz Alfaro Hospital, created and run by our renowned and unforgettable teacher Dr. Mauricio Goldenberg. I had the responsibility and the priceless honour of replacing Goldenberg in the 1970s, when he became director of the Italiano Hospital's Psychiatry Ward until his forced migration, first to Venezuela and then to the US.

It should also be noted that in his "Introduction," Carlos Nemirovsky discusses the various influences on his training and practice as a psychiatrist and psychoanalyst. The list includes not only the authors who are the focus of this book but also a great number of Argentine, US, and European thinkers. Many of them have researched and left valuable contributions to the various ways of practicing psychoanalysis and have taken political and theoretical-technical positions in the psychoanalytic field that are highlighted by Nemirovsky. Such positions allowed them to offer the benefits of psychoanalysis to the community and to numerous sectors of the population that did not have access to private psychoanalytic treatment.

At the same time, the author points to the relevance of interdisciplinary work. This approach refers to a basic notion, inter-discipline, that has become a primary frame of reference in mental health and should be the object of our continuous attention if we wish to establish an ethical viewpoint that validates the symmetrical acknowledgment of the different disciplines involved. Furthermore, we can assert that in the realm of clinical practice, the treatment currently develops as a complex space of production of techniques that incorporate a new epistemological perspective. Based on this notion, we can implement complementarities and articulations that will boost different practices as well as the diversity of psychoanalytic therapeutic strategies in mental health care, with a special effort to tackle so-called severe mental pathologies, which are designated as "complex disorders" in the title of this volume.

This special interest of Nemirovsky arose at the beginning of his training as a psychiatry resident and as a member of our ward's professional team. Like him, many of the professionals who trained at the Aráoz Alfaro hospital are currently prestigious specialists; they are practicing psychiatrists and analysts, teachers, and researchers. All of them freely opted for different psychoanalytic schools as their area of theoretical interest and chose to develop an array of forms of knowledge that make up the wide field of mental health care. We can also trace in this book the author's identification with a graduate training model that developed both the basic elements of a creative form of community mental health care and the basic premises of the concept of subjectivity and of the clinical practices of individual, family, group, institutional, and community psychotherapy in the public health system.

We should highlight here the author's references to his personal life and to his evolution in his quest to understand the vicissitudes of the human psyche. He tells us that in his hometown of Rosario, more specifically, in the town of Pérez, where he grew up in a large family, in an environment that framed "loves, passions, and rivalries but also (...) wants," he learned to survive, "and it had to be there, in that 'breeding ground,' where my psychoanalytic vocation emerged when I was a child." Beginning with this story, the text conveys to us very private aspects of Nemirovsky's waking life and even more intimate aspects of his dream activity, in a rhetorical style that recalls Freud's discourse (which appears often in the book through quotes from this author's vast work).

I will also take the liberty to disclose that readers will be pleased with the author's honesty and with his stories about his professional development and clinical practice, as well as with the comprehensive list of his personal reference points: friends, colleagues, and those who, as his teachers or analysts, left a mark on his way of thinking and facilitated his freedom of expression. In his own words,

> While my intention is to make of this book a guiding text rather than a treatise, I am content with expressing my (perhaps too personal) opinions with the hope that they will represent the views of many colleagues

who share this perspective. My goal is to transmit, in a somewhat organized way, the ideas I discuss in the courses and seminars I teach. These ideas reflect the path I have travelled, and with them I aim to help those who are starting or who have already embarked on their professional journey.

Among the issues addressed with obvious courage, it is worth mentioning Nemirovsky's comments about the genocidal military dictatorship that governed Argentina between 1976 and 1983 and about its destructive effects on public life, on the population's mental health, on institutions, and on the sociocultural milieu. At a different level, but also from a critical thinking position, he states, among other things, his views on the question of power as it arises in the patient-analyst relationship and in psychoanalytic institutions. In this context, he discusses training analysis, which has long been prescribed by the International Psychoanalytic Association, of which we are both members.

Along the path thoroughly charted by this book, readers will explore, together with the author, "Donald W. Winnicott and Heinz Kohut's basic ideas on psychic development." In his historical reference to Freud's work, Nemirovsky, who knows this work in depth, finds the original conceptual framework that is essential to our discipline. Perhaps due to his expert knowledge of Freud's texts, he goes back to them time and time again to emphasize post-Freudian contributions, especially Winnicott and Kohut's, to which he adheres both theoretically and technically, and those of other analysts who have inspired him. We can, therefore, assert that this text was conceived and carefully written to be "useful to the clinical practice of psychoanalysts, psychotherapists, and psychiatrists, especially those working with severely disturbed patients."

It is in the setting of these goals that we perceive an inspiration and desire that evoke those of many renowned psychoanalysts who are part of a long list of expert authors quoted by Nemirovsky. This list evinces the author's erudition as well as his meticulous and continued devotion to the study of the works of very diverse thinkers. He also describes the foundations of his own practice and the ideas stemming from his clinical experience. Among these ideas, history and context have become topics of particular interest that are repeatedly addressed from different conceptual perspectives.

Another key aspect of this book is the analysis of early psychic development through concepts that are common to Winnicott and Kohut yet from each of these authors' unique viewpoint. In the same way, Nemirovsky focuses on the complexity of the notions of self and narcissism, and on relational and intersubjective psychoanalysis. The author centres his discussion on the relevance of the *environment* in the constitution of the human psyche and, obviously, in the understanding of so-called psychic normalcy and pathology, in particular, those pathologies that are usually designated as severe mental disorders. When tackling these complex problems, Nemirovsky provides the broadest and most detailed theoretical-clinical references on Winnicott and Kohut's productions.

To conclude this brief prologue, it is worth pointing out that the author calls into question "orthodox" approaches to psychoanalytic practice. Throughout the book, moreover, he reveals himself as a thinker who promotes dialogue on a broad array of transcendent matters from the viewpoint of his own conceptual framework and his "unorthodox" clinical practice. In this way, he fosters a constructive discussion that will expertly enrich debates on psychoanalytic theory, training, and practice.

Barcelona, December 2018.

Note

1 Honorary Professor, Buenos Aires University; Consulting Professor, Lanus National University; Member, Argentine Psychoanalytic Association (APA), Buenos Aires Psychoanalytic Association (APdeBA), Argentine Psychoanalytic Society (SAP).

Introduction
My personal context

Authors with different views about psychoanalytic clinical practice have formulated an array of hypotheses about the development of the psyche. Each author and each school advance their own model (perspective) to understand and explain the early phenomena of psychic life that will influence adult mental organization. Original psychoanalytic theories – those that offer new ways of understanding by way of original paradigmatic ideas – prioritize specific elements, to which they grant a central role in the construction of the psyche.

Throughout this book, I have tried to develop tools to understand the formation of the adult psychic structure from the point of view of several authors with whom I have engaged in a dialogue for more than two decades. These points of view are intertwined with my personal and professional history. The favoured interlocutor of the past few years has been Winnicott, whom I consider a model for deep, independent psychoanalytic thinking. He always relied on common sense and chose a language that made his contributions accessible to a lay audience interested in the topics he discussed.

Another author who is part of my oft-consulted bibliography is Heinz Kohut, whose paradigms reformulated North American psychoanalysis. His major work is *The Restoration of the Self* (1977), where he provides an original description of the time and place where psychoanalysis was created – late-nineteenth-century Vienna. He discusses the social values that prevailed at the time, as well as his conception of the self as containing an epigenetic psyche that emerges from the relationship between individuals and their environment. It is here that Kohut's departure from the classic Freudian theory of instinct and defence (conflict theory) is clearly set formulated. The motivational focus is no longer on the sex instinct, which becomes one more factor rather than the main driving force of the human psyche. This perspective has configured its own line of research within our discipline and is currently defined as Self Psychology.

In 1981, *The International Journal of Psychoanalysis* published Kohut's posthumous paper "Introspection, empathy, and the semicircle of mental health." Against the Oedipus myth (which underlies the Freudian theory of conflict), Kohut sets up the myth of Odysseus, based on a reparatory narcissism that leads to the preservation and care of children and to inter-generational cooperation (and not necessarily to Oedipal rivalry). From this perspective, the death of Laius (a rival father) in the hands of Oedipus, as well as the later pairing of Oedipus with his mother and his consequent guilt and blindness, is *the result* of early abandonment – of the suffering of an immature self that is incapable of controlling its instincts.

In agreement with Winnicott, Kohut prioritizes the human environment and its interaction with a baby that has a strong need for its earliest objects, for its caregivers to develop its psyche (as Balint would say, it needs its objects as much as it needs air to breathe and survive). For these authors, the narcissistic needs of the human creature precede, both logically and chronologically, the organization of desire. They highlight those features of the object that allow it to satisfy the baby's elemental needs. As a result, the Freudian concept of narcissism is considerably transformed, as we shall see later. Kohut (1977) fought against the prejudice that saw narcissism as primitive and object relations as more evolved, a bias that implied that the cure depended on the transformation of narcissism into object libido to achieve maturity. Instead, he postulated two independent and equally important lines of development, namely, the development of narcissism, on the one hand, and the development of instincts and objects, on the other.

I also rely on Balint, in particular, on his notion of basic lack, as well as on Bowlby's views on attachment and McDougall's clinical developments, which I discuss later. I adopted the ideas of these cherished authors as I evolved professionally in different contexts. When I started training as a psychiatrist, Henri Ey's books were always there, and Glenn Gabbard's essays were added later on. When I became an analyst, I drew on the concepts developed by the extremely productive Argentine psychoanalytic milieu. I learned about psychoanalysis from a local perspective under the influence of Pichon-Rivière, Bleger, M. and W. Baranger, Liberman, Etchegoyen, and Gioia. Based on this blend of ideas, I tried to write a book that would be useful to the clinical practice of psychoanalysts, psychotherapists, and psychiatrists, especially those working with severely disturbed patients.

Today, psychotherapy and psychiatry, along with psychoanalysis, are my daily instruments. With them I try to give meaning to my work, to my way of being in the world. I practice psychiatry by relying on psychoanalytic concepts. This practice is enriched not only with the writings of the authors I cited above but also, above all, with the notions developed by diverse inter-subjective perspectives, from Ferenczi on. These ideas provide a slant, a way of constructing the clinical situation, especially with severely ill patients. Experience has led me to think that severe illness – and I am not talking about diagnosis – is always complex (disorders emerge in multiple ways: in the body, at work, in the family). Therefore, we must examine it from manifold perspectives, both psychoanalytic and non-psychoanalytic.

Concerning psychiatry, this book's subtitle is likely inspired in the memorable article by Winnicott (1959), "Classification: Is There a Psychoanalytic

Contribution to Psychiatric Classification?". There, Winnicott portrays the psychiatry/psychoanalysis dialectic, which reflects his own career. The professional journey of all those who trained as resident physicians also began with the care of hospital patients, and we slowly acquired psychoanalytic knowledge.[1] At the Aráoz Alfaro Hospital we incorporated a point of view that is now completely integrated into our way of thinking and will likely never cease to be present.

I became a psychiatrist, and gradually acquired a solid psychoanalytic training. This does not mean that two separate dimensions took shape inside me or that my clinical work has operated through a schematic, crude choice between the two disciplines – "this is a psychiatric patient, this is a psychoanalytic patient." I could never separate my activities in clinical practice. I recognize myself as a psychoanalyst who does not mind being a physician and psychiatrist. I never think of helping patients by using a certain approach and excluding others; I do everything I can for them. It is later, when I discuss my work with my colleagues, that they will point out that I chose a certain perspective as a tool in a specific intervention.[2]

Sometimes I need to prescribe medication to relieve patients' symptomatic suffering and thus create better conditions for the treatment. In this way, I can form a therapeutic couple with the patient that will introduce a new relational model. To this end, I must develop a variety of psychoanalytic hypotheses based on my training, because that is my way of asking questions and of asking myself questions as a psychoanalyst. Perhaps I start with two deficits. I cannot be a psychiatrist pure and simple (if we view psychiatrists as taxonomists of mental pathologies), just as I cannot see myself at the other end of the spectrum, that is, as a psychoanalyst with no hospital experience who has never seen a psychotic person or worked in a community. My practice, therefore, necessarily travels a path that has been both enriched and constrained by my identifications with earlier and current teachers.

Another aspect of my professional vantage point that ought to be mentioned here is my inability to conceive of a practice that is not based on the evidential paradigm (Ginzburg, 1992), which I discuss later. Our ideas and our professional way of operating stem from our family and personal histories, our professional development, our socio-historical environment, and our teachers and their clinical practice. We are "doomed" to a changing history. Our "third complemental series" will be our practice, which will inevitably include our theoretical framework. Yet if we are honest with ourselves, and if we survive and are daring enough, we will discover new paths.

The general context in which we are immersed affects our perception of our professional world, and the personal theories we develop must become our slaves, not our masters, paraphrasing Guntrip (1971). While my intention is to make of this book a guiding text rather than a treatise, I am content with expressing my (perhaps too personal) opinions with the hope that they will represent the views of many colleagues who share this perspective. My goal is to transmit, in a somewhat organized way, the ideas I discuss in the courses and seminars I teach. These ideas reflect the path I have travelled, and with them I aim to help those who are starting or who have already embarked on their professional journey.

I attempted these reflections some decades after graduating from Buenos Aires University's Medical School and starting my training as a psychiatrist at a high-complexity general hospital. There, residents tried to take advantage of the various resources at our disposal: individual, group, and family psychotherapy; mass meetings with patients in "assemblies," as we called them; occupational therapy; workshops; and so on. These were the initial years of our psychiatric and psychotherapeutic practice. We engaged in endless discussions in order to reach our goal, to improve patients' mental health, although some of us were beginning to aim toward the "pure psychoanalytic cure" (a colleague of the incipient Lacanian school accused us of being mentalthealthists!). When the military coup took place in 1976, an open wound was inflicted – our psychiatry ward was gradually dismantled, and the community healthcare approach, which was our major goal, eliminated. The group lost its richness and heterogeneity, as well as its connection with the community.

Intersubjetivists rightly argue that we cannot overlook the context in which authors formulate their hypotheses. Knowing their context and biographical information helps generate empathy toward these authors. Everything is eventually present in the stories we tell. As Borges (1977, p. 21) puts it, "My story will be true to reality or, in any case, to my personal memory of reality, which amounts to the same thing." I will tell you a bit about my history, about my origins. Like everyone else, I have many origins and various myths about them. When viewed from different contexts and vital moments, these stories change me, sometimes despite myself. Our experiences, which, I am well aware, do not accumulate by apposition, give rise to new perspectives, to unprecedented ways of seeing that force us to make our constructions more complex. Historicizing also involves demystifying, denaturalizing our belief that events occur in a reassuring straight line, like a plateau. As José Bleger taught the residents in psychiatry at the Aráoz Alfaro hospital, there is no "natural history."

The current product, the person I am and the person I recognize in myself, is a combination of three inextricably linked landscapes, namely, Rosario, Lanús, and Buenos Aires. I was delivered professionally in Lanus, at the Aráoz Alfaro Hospital, but I grew up in Buenos Aires, at the Buenos Aires Psychoanalytic Association (APdeBA). Conception occurred in Rosario or, to be precise, a few kilometres from there, in Pérez, a small town where my father had built a modest weekend home in a "community" lot where five of his siblings and siblings-in-law had also built houses. We spent three or four months a year there, and what with siblings, uncles, and cousins, we were more than 30. This environment, which served as a context not only for loves, passions, and rivalries but also for wants, taught me about survival. And it had to be there, in that "breeding ground," where my psychoanalytic vocation emerged. Later, *The Interpretation of Dreams, Jokes...*, and the first medical histories came my way. At 14, these readings mingled with *The Art of Loving, Sandokan, Heart, Listen Yankee: The Revolution in Cuba,* and The Old Testament.

In the professional field, my most significant place of origin was "el Lanus," the Aráoz Alfaro Hospital (today, the Evita Hospital), a melting pot for ideas and therapeutic models that is still alive in me today, recreating itself in my memory as a possible ideal and hopeful guide rather than as a utopia. The very different leaderships of Mauricio Goldenberg[3] and (especially for me) of Valentín Barenblit created a facilitating context that, as a framework, allowed us to develop unique psychotherapeutic practices that summarized and integrated the most diverse aetiological aspects of pathologies in the manner of complemental series. Considering the complex situations of the patients we saw at the Psychiatric Ward, it was impossible not to take into account the manifold aspects involved in mental pathology. Consultations always included all the ingredients making up the mosaic of factors causing illness, causes that we schematically defined as biological, psychological, and social.

This way of looking at mental illness, taking into consideration its causal complexity, resulted in endless arguments among residents about what pathology, or what aspect of each pathology, corresponded to each of these three areas. How could we avoid reducing aetiology to what appeared to us as a single factor? If the illness had social causes, what role could or should we play as psychotherapists? If we tackled pathologies that had a clear social origin by supporting patients with psychotherapy and medication, weren't we preventing them from dealing with the problem that had originated the illness? If we were striving for consistency, shouldn't we operate on all the factors that had contributed to the pathology and expand our scope of intervention by devoting more time to social action and less to psychotherapy? Wouldn't it mean falling into a blinding trap if we concerned ourselves with the social aspects of an illness while conducting a psychotherapy, instead of focusing on the individual, or if we saw the hospital as an illusory shelter from what was taking place outside its walls?

Several generations of residents were forged in the clamour of these arguments, and we gradually understood that our patients presented with sets of symptoms that could not be easily typified. Only by forcing a classification could we claim that there were no inextricable aetiological combinations. These experiences were probably the ones that most influenced me. During my medical residency, I came into contact with Bleger, Pichon-Rivière, Liberman, Zac, and R. Paz, and also during this period, I had the pleasure of consulting on a daily basis with senior colleagues, professionals/examples who were committed to their work and their questions, such as Ricón, Fiorini, Fernández Moujan, H. Bleichmar, Sluzki, Bucahi, Kuten, and Siculer.

In the next stage in my career, at the hospital's Centre for Alcoholism (along with Ferralli and Verruno), I was faced with grimmer pathology. A few years later, after the disappearance of our dear colleague Marta Brea and the government's taking control of the ward in 1976/1977, we all scattered due to the genocidal dictatorship. With the departure of my teacher and model, Valentín Barenblit, for Barcelona, I was forced to look for an institution that could guide me in my vocation. Perhaps because of my personality, or because I needed to find a political justification for it, I could not choose an individual learning experience. I therefore sought the plurality of APdeBA. A lecture on alcoholism by Horacio Etchegoyen encouraged me to join the Association. When he finished speaking, I stayed to ask questions about my alcoholic patients, trying to take advantage of Horacio's extensive experience on this issue and his very accessible and compelling way of combining the psychiatric lexicon with psychoanalytic concepts.

Patiently enduring the onslaught of questions, he generously invited me to supervise with him for free, and made time to see me. The behaviour of this paradigmatic teacher, supporting and generous, who was studying a pathology that, due to its prevalence in Argentina's marginalized populations, was being overlooked, filled me with gratitude. Based on my experience with Etchegoyen, I transferred my trust to APA's Ateneo group, which was the precursor of APdeBA, and requested a training analyst. Horacio suggested Roberto Polito, who became my analyst and provided me with a unique experience.

I was part of the second group of candidates at APdeBA's Psychoanalytic Institute. Courses and supervisions did their job. Near the end of my fourth year of classes, I started undergoing what I call *the turn*. My training was essentially Freudian and Kleinian. When I presented a clinical vignette in one of my classes, my professor, an excellent clinician, asked me about my frame of reference. I answered that I could not define it. I simply thought I should act the way I was acting, but I was not taking theory into account – I did not even know which authors could justify my decision. My answer greatly displeased my teacher, who advised that I go back to my readings and adopt a clear frame of reference instead of "operating like a hybrid."

I tried to follow his advice but found that my readings at the Institute, my readings as a resident, and my identification figures (among them, Barenblit, H. Bleichmar, and other ideals from the early stages of my career, such as Ricón, Fiorini, and Slutzki) formed such an intricate landscape that I could not see myself reflected in a "clear frame of reference." From then on, I started to accept (while making sure my professor did not notice) that my "modality" was this mix (which, far from being eclectic, gradually changed as I studied and acquired more experience). Such combination of viewpoints has very much enhanced my ability to understand and probably help my patients.

At that time, after immersing ourselves in Freud, we studied Kleinian and post-Kleinian ideas intensively and in depth. Other authors were discussed only in a few courses. I have psychoanalytic "grandparents" and "parents" whom I take after: Balint, Winnicott, Kohut, Ferenczi, Fairbairn, and Mahler, among the foreigners, and among ours, Polito, Liberman, Bleger, Gioia, Painceira, Lancelle, and Valeros have become examples who embody new ideas. Nonetheless, as usually happens with today's children, I probably resemble my contemporaries (my "siblings") more than my parents – those siblings who are my training peers, my friends, and who have accompanied me in my writing, research, and teaching adventures. I would like to name some of them: Spivacow, Alba, Zonis, Aguilar, Bricht, Seiguer, Ferrali, R. Moguillansky, M. Nemirovsky, Paulucci, Abello, A. Liberman, M. Fernandez Depetris, R. Rojas Jerez, and M. Milchberg. And I surely try to resemble those I passionately read today: Mitchell, Green, H. Bleichmar, Stolorow, McDougall, Killingmo, Renik, Bollas, Benjamin, Aron, Pitzer, Slochower, Borgogno, and Orange.

The turn toward the authors who have become my current reference points was prompted by the treatment of an adult borderline patient who was besieged by a variety of symptoms, each as acute as the next: anxiety, hypochondria of different kinds, conversions, tics, rituals. Furthermore, she would every now and then present with fainting, rage, and other kinds of fits during which she would bang her head against the wall or attack herself by cutting or biting herself. Her partner was a schizoid man who reported feeling bewildered and overwhelmed by her and who, as a way out (that is what he called it) and to "save his skin," had gotten a job in the provinces. He travelled for days at a time, leaving the patient alone.

At times she was calm, and it was then that she was able to examine things in depth and to commit herself to her therapy. Yet when she broke down, she did so in full colour, triggering a chain reaction. During her first visits to my office, she would jump from the couch to the bathroom and then would bang her head against the wall or slam the door to show her anger against me, or would parody me derisively. I had to refit my office so that she would not get hurt, and forbid her to open doors leading to private places or take out objects that she would threaten to throw at me. As much as I tried, I could not understand the process of her illness based on the theoretical framework I had developed back then.

After two years of treatment in the style that was customary at the time (on the couch, when she was able to recline on it, and four sessions a week during more than ten months of the year), she started calling me at home at night and sometimes in the early hours of the morning to hear my voice. "I want to hear you speak, that's all," she would say to me. Once I had uttered some words, whatever I was able to say, she would calm down and would be able to endure (that is how I saw it) the time that must elapse until the next session. I was surprised that I did not perceive her calls as violent irruptions (the way my supervisor understood them). I always felt that her attempt to communicate responded to her need to maintain a link with me, which time dissolved. She needed to get back in touch, even if by phone.

Interpretations following the line suggested by my supervisor (which pointed to her intrusion into my private life or to her attacks on the love relationship she fantasized I had) did not take root in me; I saw them as foreign and, therefore, heard myself voicing them in an unconvincing way. I insisted on underscoring her invasion of my privacy only to fail repeatedly.

It was then that I asked Alfredo Painceira to become my supervisor and started avidly reading the bibliography he recommended. During this new stage of the treatment I was able to understand that the patient was expressing a demand in an environment that was very different from the one where she had grown up, perhaps for the first time in her life, to a listener who was trying to understand her. This demand constituted an attempt to establish a hopeful, successful bond, unlike the early relationships in which she had participated as a child and as a young woman.

I felt much more responsible for her reactions (which I gradually understood as a response to our separations) and stopped interpreting her aggression as projective identification. I maintained our connection without blaming her. I understood that she was aggressive or "came apart" because she was very frightened, that she felt lonely and helpless, and started to realize that my tone of voice, my calm waiting attitude, and historical construction, rather than transference interpretations, allowed me to create valuable moments during which she was capable of reflection. Thanks to her thoughts, I could assemble sequences from her past history and her present that gave meaning to her fits of rage and hypochondriac symptoms, which we understood as her response to threats of helplessness.

This experience drove me to study my patients with new tools and to recognize paradoxical clinical phenomena, such as those we see in our consulting rooms today. During those years I acknowledged that my own discipline did not provide enough instruments to understand processes that are very common among our patients. I was lucky to contact Marta López Gil, who opened my eyes to the context of social ties in which we are immersed. Later it was Marta Zatonyi who, from the perspective of art history, guided me in the complex reading of Nietzsche, Heiddeger, and the contemporary hermeneutics scholars (Ricoeur, Gadamer, Vattimo, and Rorty) who have enriched our thinking.

Today, I see that many of my patients are beset by uncertainty and superficiality and are trying to survive with the inconsistency of their being. They are removed from the classic symptomatic structuring of desire and defences, and hence incapable of benefiting from traditional psychoanalysis. Many decades have passed between Freud's "hysterics" and today's narcissists, and between the notion of a closed psychic apparatus governed by drives and aiming to release and the intersubjective construction posited by Mitchell, Lyons-Ruth, Aron, Renik, Stolorow, and Atwood (among the most renowned intersubjectivists). During these years, authors have posited an evolving subjectivity typical of our times that greatly differs from the Central European subjectivity described more than a century ago. Even if they still seem radical to me, these hypotheses are probably the meeting point between my present and future way of thinking.

Just as I tell readers where I come from, I should also mention where I am going on the institutional path. There are some things I know about my journey. I have always considered that the psychoanalytic institution is indispensable for our professional training and development, but it took me some time to become a training analyst despite having the necessary credentials. I do not believe that candidates' training analysis should meet current institutional requirements. A good analysis that is accepted by the association to which the candidate belongs should be enough. We should turn back to Guntrip (1975, p. 145), who wonders somewhat ironically: "How complete a result did our own training analysis produce?"

This analysis involves a complex relationship between psychoanalysis and power. I am not talking about power in the sense of subjection to certain ideas or persons, but about the power that training analysts necessarily wield, regardless of their attitude, just by belonging to an institution that sees this device as essential for the transformation of a candidate into an analyst. Analysis is indispensable for analytic training; it is likely the most important of the pillars making up the training tripod (personal analysis, supervision, and classes). Nevertheless, the link between the institution and the training analyst draws a boundary between the members of the therapeutic couple – an obstacle that is hard to tackle from inside the relationship. Many of us refer patients to analysts who may or may not be training analysts. We do so very carefully, and may later verify the benefits or lack thereof of these analyses, their processes and results. Why should we consider a candidate's analytic treatment differently?

Today I believe that setting institutional rules for an analysis does not necessarily benefit our training, and as the Spanish singer-songwriter Joan Manuel Serrat might say, I'd rather have an analysis than a training analysis, or a good analysis than one that has been systematized by an institution.[4] Regarding the definition of "complete" questioned by Guntrip, in my view, due to the way training analysis is established, it will inevitably be incomplete, regardless of the characteristics of the therapeutic couple. This is particularly true because, due to the features of this type of analysis, it is difficult to examine the power relations involved. The institution associated with the analytic training will generate indirect countertransferences, and will also be present in the perspective of both participants. Such presence of institutional power may become, I believe, a bastion (Baranger and Baranger, 2008) hard to avoid.

Notes

1 We identified as dynamic psychiatrists. The addition of this "last name" distinguished us from so-called traditional psychiatrists. Yet when we finished our residency, the Ministry of Health awarded us the title of Psychopathology Resident (sic), which means that in the eyes of the official power at that time we were not "true psychiatrists." This old debate is still ongoing. In this sense, Ey (1977) starts his book *En defensa de la psiquiatría* (Defence and Illustration of Psychiatry) by saying that

> psychiatry is medical or it is not (...) notwithstanding the views of those who criticize it for being too much so, and had rather it were 'moral,'

'anthropological,' 'social,' or even 'political' (that is, nothing at all) and forego to take mental health as their true object in the specific reality of its psychopathological structure.

(Ey, 1977, p. 14)

Gabbard (2005) has a different approach. He titles his book *Psychodynamic Psychiatry in Clinical Practice*, and states in his preface that psychodynamic psychiatry "must be regarded today as situated within the overarching construct of *biopsychosocial* psychiatry" (Gabbard, 2005, p. 4; author's emphasis). Without dismissing Ey's extraordinary merits, I find myself closer to Gabbard's position.

2 Just as when I was a child I was put to the test by being confronted with a dilemma that, as such, was impossible to solve when I was repeatedly asked the question, "Are you Jewish or Argentine?", now I often encounter someone at a social gathering who will blurt out, "Are you a psychiatrist or a psychoanalyst?" This question is often accompanied by another one: "Do you use a couch or drugs?" These questions always puzzle me. A few years ago I tried to explain to my interlocutor that these concepts were not mutually exclusive. Today, I think that the person asking the question does not really want to know the answer, and if we attempt to offer one, it will likely be boring to them.

3 R. Moguillansky (1992) argues that

Goldenberg should be credited with the establishment of the first Psychopathology Ward in a general hospital and the setting in motion of what was probably the most serious social psychiatry program ever implemented in this country. He promoted the most significant research project in the epidemiology of mental health to be carried out in the Buenos Aires Metropolitan Area. He made relevant contributions to the organization and planning of mental healthcare in the entire Latin American region. He opened a significant path in the Department of Psychiatry of Buenos Aires University's Medical School, which became a reference point for those interested in a mental healthcare that did not opt for asylums (...) Besides being personally indebted to him, APdeBA [Buenos Aires Psychoanalytic Association] members acknowledge how much psychoanalysis owes to him (...) he helped test our instrument in the treatment of severe pathologies and put it in contact with interdisciplinary studies. Thanks to him, psychoanalysis expanded not only toward the treatment of more severe pathologies, but also to reach low-income sectors.

(Moguillansky, 1992, no pagination)

4 The author alludes to the song "*Cada loco con su tema*" [To each his own], where Serrat gives a long list of preferences that include "roads to borders / a butterfly to Rockefeller Centre (...) kissing to laughing, / dancing to parading..." (T. N.).

1 Early psychic development after Freud[1]

...it would be pleasant if we were to be able to take for analysis only those patients whose mothers at the very start and also in the first months had been able to provide good-enough conditions. But this era of psycho-analysis is steadily drawing to a close.

Winnicott (1955, pp. 290–291)

...in contrast to the personality structure of the fin de siècle patients whose investigation led Freud to his formulation of the dichotomized psyche and later of structural conflict, the prevalent personality organization of our time is not typified by the simple horizontal split brought about by repression. The psyche of modern man – the psyche described by Kafka and Proust and Joyce – is enfeebled, multifragmented (vertically split), and disharmonious. It follows that we cannot adequately understand our patients and explain them to themselves if we try to do so with the aid of a model of unconscious conflicts that cannot do the job.

Kohut (1984, p. 60)

The temporal context

This chapter discusses approaches[2] derived from Winnicott and Kohut's basic ideas on psychic development. Many of the formulations advanced by Winnicott, in particular, had been addressed earlier or contemporarily by prolific analytic thinkers such as Fairbairn and Bowlby, and especially by Ferenczi. These earlier thinkers postulated similar approaches. Yet due to a variety of reasons that would be worth exploring in our search for our origin as analysts, their viewpoints did not consolidate as schools of psychoanalytic thought until the advent of the authors who are the focus of this book.[3]

Elsewhere, I argue that

since the death of the founder of psychoanalysis, our discipline has undergone considerable shifts that are largely the product of the cultural transformation of analysands and analysts. We have witnessed the birth and development of mutations that have challenged basic paradigms.

Slowly, our way of thinking (psychoanalytic theory) and of operating in the session (psychoanalytic technique) have changed.

(Nemirovsky, 1993 p. 2)

Etchegoyen (1991), for his part, states that if we "take a bird's eye view of how the psychoanalytic science has evolved, we are faced with a clear-cut dividing line that coincides with the end of Freud's life" (Etchegoyen, 1991, p. 88). Nevertheless, choosing 1939 as our starting point could certainly be biased or arbitrary, since some strong schools of thought were developing before then that challenged basic aspects of psychoanalysis and gave rise to fiery debates (Jung, Adler, and Ferenczi's reformulations constitute highlights in the history of our discipline). Even so, we must acknowledge that the years of World War II are highly significant. From the 1940s on, some of the paradigms of the psychoanalytic "schools" that can be identified today were beginning to take shape.

Green (1975) also points out that "since Freud's death, and doubtless even before that, one can no longer refer to psychoanalytic theory in the singular" (1986 [1997], p. 13). The history of psychoanalysis always involved debate, and this debate enriched theories and techniques. In this sense, among the milestones that populate the first half of the twentieth century are the founder's controversies with Jung, Adler, Rank, and Steckel, and later with Ferenczi. There are also the British School's innovations concerning the analysis of children and psychotic patients, spearheaded by Jones and Klein, as well as the latter's debate with Anna Freud. These were followed by the original evolution of psychoanalysis in the US with Hartmann, Kris, and Lowenstein, and later, back in Europe, by Lacan's novel concepts.

If we go further back in time, we should keep in mind that Freud's first ideas emerged in authoritarian Victorian society, whose basic values guided his research. These values were the discovery of truth and the achievement of psychological individuality (Kohut, 1984). In the same way, it is worth highlighting that in the last years of Freud's work, as Erikson ([1982] 1997, p. 22) points out,

> the historical period in which we learned to observe such revelations of the inner life was well on its way to turning into one of the most catastrophic periods in history; and the ideological division between the 'inner-' and the 'outerworld' may well have had deep connotations of a threatening split between the individualistic enlightenment rooted in Judaeo-Christian civilization and the totalitarian veneration of the racist state.

Science based on positivism,[4] which inherited the enlightenment's viewpoint, had its most conspicuous representatives in Darwin, Pasteur, Koch, Lister, and Curie; in pragmatists such as Peirce; and, in the transition into the twentieth century, in Russell, Bohr, and Einstein (to name a few). These authors also constituted reference points and, doubtlessly, a valuable guide for Freud in his choice of methodology for the new discipline. In this sense, Freud had to interact with two opposite historical developments. These were the prevalence of scientific methods derived from the natural sciences (which excluded anything that could not be grasped through objectification and measurement), and the irruption of subjectivism and its gradual domination over the cultural world (the end of Romanticism and the emergence of Impressionism and later of Surrealism).

In the Central Europe of his time, Freud's cultural education blended Victorian values with his family's and his personal values. From this perspective, he laid the foundations of the analytic method based on his self-analysis (ultimately, the analysis of an adult male who had not experienced major suffering) and the analysis of his patients, also adults. In the heart of Hapsburg Vienna, working, like every late-nineteenth-century professional, in his own home surrounded by his family, Freud started to delve into the human psyche, the Oedipus complex, childhood sexuality, psychic reality, and the formation of systems or agencies and of complexes or structures. This happened 100 years ago.

It should not seem strange to us, then, that practitioners of psychoanalysis, whose creator, in this particular juncture, was fervently seeking the truth rather than the confirmation of established dogmas, would reformulate many of the founder's viewpoints as the discipline evolved. Paraphrasing Guntrip (1971), Freud set down the cornerstone but did not build the entire building. Cultural expressions (fine arts, architecture, and poetry) always integrate axiological changes taking place in the society where they originate. Thus, early-nineteenth-century architecture in Vienna reflected a centripetal everyday life. Focus on the home facilitated the development of an extremely stimulating family life.[5] Today's family life, by contrast, shows a very strong centrifugal tendency and takes place in buildings whose inhabitants are anonymous.

Back then, the social climate favoured the development of the "prima donna" of the early twentieth century, hysteria, which always needs presences. As a consequence, the first analysts focused on what would obviously attract their attention – the Oedipus complex and its by-product, neurosis. Based on their clinical practice, they could explain this pathology's origin and evolution and formulate narrow working explanations that were consistent with the scientific methodologies of the time. They created a metapsychology for neurosis, and, therefore, nascent psychoanalysis could not encompass those clinical pictures that remained outside this psychopathology.

Today, schizoid and borderline pathologies, born from failed encounters and separations (and feeding on absences), have displaced hysteria from its favored position and require new explanations that will contemplate present-day family and social organizations, that is, that will take the environment into account as a necessary factor. With an empathic effort, which contemporary historians deem necessary to understand our past (Carr,

1967), we can grasp many of Freud's reasons for anxiety when conducting his first investigations. As we mentioned earlier, this anxiety arose from an attempt to place psychoanalysis within the natural sciences by resorting to the appropriate lexicon, which included words such as cathexis, psychic apparatus, and libido.

Today, almost no one would include our discipline among the exact sciences. Our method is closer to historical research, to narrative than to the methods of the so-called natural sciences. We start from history (the history of a patient, a family, a group), and from there we hypothesize the context of our clinical inquiry. We are constantly asking what this history is, what it is leaving out, and how to narrow it. We often wonder, what then is history? The tautology that defines it as what historians do (same as defining psychoanalysis as what psychoanalysts do) underscores the difficulty in finding clear paradigms to frame our work. Historians and analysts use provisional, junctural, temporary criteria that are based on traces, documents, narratives ... Can we try to be more precise, for now, without running the risk of using definitions that are unfairly exclusive?

We know that history is never homogeneous or unidirectional. Nor does it respond to the action-reaction principle – to simple, mechanical facts. Historians have to deal with opinions and pressure. Some attempt to homogenize data; the creators of so-called historical truth think they gain by writing texts that reflect "the official story." We often find that it is the owners of this truth who believe they have won and who usually write the history texts. In this sense, one of the issues we must address is how we define *fact* in our discipline. Significant facts, those narrated by the author, are obviously interpretations of what took place. Furthermore, we call them *facts* because they are psychologically active, effective, and have an effect of truth, of reality, of having happened.

I would like to go back to Carr (1961), who quotes Professor Sir George Clark. In referring to historians "of a later generation," Clark points out that these historians "consider that knowledge of the past has come down through one or more human minds (...) and therefore cannot consist of elemental and impersonal atoms which nothing can alter" (Carr, 1961, p. 3). We know that there is no objective historical truth, that the so-called material truth is not a topic of analysis. We must, therefore, view facts as accepted judgements that resemble an event that took place. History, after all, is the history of thought, and it implies a certain perspective – the historian's perspective, which is in consonance with its context.

This reconstruction of the past in the mind of historians/psychoanalysts relies on what is, for them, empirical evidence. Yet their evidence is not a mere list of data. Rather, the process of reconstruction is governed by the selection and interpretation of facts. It is this process that makes them, precisely, historical facts. In psychoanalysis, selection and interpretation resorts to clues instead of evidence. In my view, clues are more valuable for our work than mere statistics or the enumeration of the obvious (Ginzburg,

1992). From this perspective, then, we understand that the primary task of historians (or psychoanalysts) is not to collect but to assess, to collect while assessing, because if we do not assess, how can we identify material that deserves to be collected?

It should not sound odd to us what has been said so often about history, that is, that historical facts do not exist for historians ... until they themselves create them. Ricoeur (1977) claims that psychoanalytic theory selects and codifies facts within the context of the analytic session, and that these facts are mediated by language and addressed to others. They are not necessarily observable but result from the meaning that events acquire for patients – the same events that psychotherapists consider from the position of observer. Ricoeur examines psychoanalytic facts in four dimensions: they can be narrated; they are addressed to others; they are fantasized, figured, or symbolized; and they are collected in the narrative of a biography (historicized). This author coincides with Habermas's analysis regarding the separation between historical-hermeneutic sciences (sciences of the spirit that respond to practical interest and are regulated by intersubjectivity) and sciences that aspire to objectivity.

Guntrip (1967), based on Home (1966), suggests that psychoanalysis is the study of the subjective experiences of living objects by way of a subjective, internal process that we call recognition or understanding of our immediate experience. At the same time, Benedetto Croce's contribution teaches us that history is always contemporary history; we can only grasp something of the past through the lens of the present, in light of the problems and needs of the current context. Then, is history a biased perspective? If we look at how we see the Middle Ages today and how they were seen during the Renaissance, we will probably find that the selected facts are completely different.[6]

If we asked what Freud represents to contemporary analysts (setting aside those analysts who, due to their narcissistic bond with the master, have turned his theory into dogma via idealization), we can agree on the paradigm of the tireless, non-conformist, and enthusiastic researcher who theorizes and then refutes himself. As a consequence, his scientific work is always open and is neither uniform nor linear. If we adopt a healthy perspective, we will be able to identify with his curiosity, his scientific rigour, and his openness to the new. After all, he would say that the only sacred text is the patient's, and patients are never the same – there are new pathologies, prevalence varies, we "construct" different patients in different cultures. Today we can rebut, supplement, or decentre the result of many of Freud's inquiries, but his method (his way of doing research) will likely remain almost unchanged.[7]

According to Green,

mourning Freud means that we are forced to realize:

1. that he is no longer here to continue to rectify his work according to the teachings of clinical practice, as he used to do; 2. that even if he were

here, he would be useless to us because he would continue to think like a man from the early twentieth century; 3. that neither can we fail to notice that his genius did not free him from remaining blind to certain realities or from being permeated by an ideology that must be challenged; 4. that none of Freud's successors, aside from some utterly outstanding contributions, offers a replacement solution; 5. that we must manage on our own, taking a critical perspective – a perspective that is critical of Freud's work from the inside, and critical of Freud's work from the outside, that is, according to our experience and our epistemology.

(Green, 1996, p. 224)

When we tell our story, relying on the past but from the perspective of the present, we always talk about a movement ... everything happens in a process ("going on being," as Winnicott calls it, resorting to the present continuous to signify an uninterrupted process of "gradually becoming"). The work of the main authors discussed in this book spread across the psychoanalytic world after World War II. Winnicott published articles that, rooted in his experience, prioritized environmental factors in the constitution of the early psyche (Winnicott, 1945, 1952, 1956). Somewhat later, Kohut (1959, 1966) advocated the reassessment of narcissism (which was viewed at the time as developed on the basis of early object relations and as lacking in significance) as a "driving force" of the psyche.

Their occupying important positions in their respective institutions and their administrative work at the national and international levels facilitated the dissemination of these authors' ideas. Winnicott presided the British Psychoanalytic Association twice, and Kohut was president of the North American Psychoanalytic Association and vice president of the International Psychoanalytical Association. Holding these positions granted political power to their scientific ideas. Today we can see how these perspectives, new ways of conceiving the psyche, had a multiplying effect. Many thinkers have been able to play with them in a creative way by confronting them, combining the two or each of them with other authors' perspectives, or following the paths they opened to develop their own.

It would be hard to draw a boundary between the adherents to each of these authors' ideas. In the first generation we may highlight the work of Khan, Laing, Milner, Gaddini, and Bollas, who followed in Winnicott's steps. Kohut's successors, for their part, followed in his with different approaches. We should mention authors such as Gedo, Orstein, Orange, Bacal, Stolorow, Goldberg, Mitchell, Branchasft, and Lichtenberg, whose ideas configured true schools (we can talk about first-topography Kohutians, relationalists, intersubjectivists, and other schools that are still developing). Other contemporaries, such as McDougall and Green, did not join any school but drew directly from Winnicott and Kohut or from related sources, and contributed to the current development of psychoanalysis with their own theories.

It is worth recalling here Guntrip's famous quote: "Theory (...) is a useful servant but a bad master, liable to produce orthodox defenders of every variety of the faith" (Guntrip, 1975, p. 145). Nonetheless, we know (based on clinical experience) that our theory will often become our master, and that it is utopic, or naïve, to posit, as did Wallerstein (1988), that analysts have in clinical theory a common, unifying element. Guntrip's own perspective does not seem very flexible. Strong adhesions (analysts' identities concerning their Weltanschauung) appear to be unavoidable, and constitute a resistance or bastion in our work with patients. Perhaps this is one of the main reasons why we need to open psychoanalysis to a dialogue with other disciplines. If we increase the surfaces of contact during psychoanalytic training, maybe we will avoid the easy temptation to have a single master.

Some post-Freudian contributions to early psychic development

Traditionally (Cvik, 1984), analysts considered as early psychic development the infantile sexual development that lasted till the culmination of the Oedipus complex, and called this period the child's "prehistory." This perspective defined development based on the evolution of instincts. Before Winnicott and Kohut, there were only marginal references to the role of the environment.

Authors such as Mahler, Winnicott, and Kohut stress that primitive development takes place exclusively in the mother-baby matrix. As we shall see later, Winnicott states that the baby does not exist as a separate entity and emphatically asserts that we cannot distinguish the child from the maternal figure. As Lancelle puts it,

in the first stages, abstracting the infant from this undifferentiated matrix and talking about a child as a distinct being (with drives, fantasies, intentionality, and so on) is a resource of questionable usefulness that is dangerously exposed to adultomorphic deformations.

(Lancelle, 1984, p. 453)

From the beginning of life, the baby needs objects that will hold it, handle it, and facilitate its gradual approach to the object world (Winnicott), that will mirror it and allow idealized fusion so that it will feel safe (Kohut). If these objects, embodied in the maternal figure (who is not necessarily the baby's biological mother), respond to these needs, they will ensure the continuity of the developing self without traumatic effractions. Their emphasis on the specific response of environmental objects is what characterizes these authors' approach. If the atmosphere surrounding the baby is unhealthy, we will find the consequences in our practice. If the environment repeatedly fails to respond appropriately, we shall be dealing with deficit pathologies.

Why is the focus displaced from instinct and its transformations to bonding modes? Why do these perspectives decentre the Oedipal knot as the cornerstone of mental pathology and direct the gaze to those aspects of the link that precede triangular organization? Let us consider the contextual starting point of our authors' theory and practice. Winnicott, Kohut, and some of their contemporaries were concerned with the individual produced by the urban environment, and this concern is obviously reflected in their inquiries. Many forms of post-war psychological suffering were a consequence of humans' inability to find the other's presence, availability, and understanding, to have instances of meeting, and to enjoy intergenerational cooperation and respect for one's intimacy, values that are much less relevant at the height of post-industrial society than they were during Freudian modernity.

In their need to formulate hypotheses about origin, psychoanalytic researchers have always developed more or less complex theories about the birth of the psyche. The psychoanalytic method, which aims to trace a backward path through patients' history, usually tries to reach the earliest moment in that history, which varies for each school. For Winnicott (1967a), early and deep are not synonymous; he draws a clear distinction between what comes first chronologically (the as-yet undifferentiated environment of the subject) and what lies deepest in the psyche (aspects tied to depressive phenomena and hatred). Early events, then, tend not to be part of the self, although they are part of the subject's history. They constitute what the environment gave the baby during the first stages of extrauterine life in terms of holding, handling, and object-presenting. Deep elements, in turn, are gradually incorporated as content of the self.

If there were deficiencies in the environment of the baby right after birth that gave rise to a traumatic situation, the effects would probably appear in the context of an analysis as "need transferences" (Lerner and Nemirovsky, 1989b). Such transferences are often solved by the setting and the para-interpretive aspects of the analyst's activity (presence, tone and pitch, and actions). Deep aspects will emerge as long as we enable resolution by facilitating the reparation of early failures.

On the concept of the self

I will only highlight some ideas tied to the notion of the self that are close to the conception of the authors discussed here. Hence, I will not dwell on the first contributions to this concept made by Hartman, Jacobson, Mahler, and Kernberg. Stern (1985, pp. 5–7) writes that the self and its boundaries "are at the heart of philosophical speculation on human nature" and that the sense of self and other may be found across cultures and bears great influence on every social experience. No matter how many differing views there are on what the self actually is, claims Stern, adult human beings have "a very real sense of self that permeates daily social experience." This author outlines a variety of perceptions of the self: as "a single, distinct, integrated body"; as the agent of acts; as the entity that experiences feelings; as the agency that defines our intentions; as the planner, the speaker, "the communicator and sharer of personal knowledge."

We are usually unaware of these senses of self, "but they can be brought to and held in consciousness. We instinctively process our experiences in such a way that they appear to belong to some kind of unique subjective organization that we commonly call the sense of self." While we seem to be unable to determine its nature, our sense of self "stands as an important subjective reality, a reliable, evident phenomenon that the sciences cannot dismiss. How we experience ourselves in relation to others provides a basic organizing perspective for all interpersonal events." Stern also argues that some of these senses of self precede both self-awareness and language. These are "the senses of agency, of physical cohesion, of continuity in time, of having intentions in mind...".

We should recall here that in his introduction to *The Ego and the Id*, Strachey points out that we can identify two major uses of '*das Ich*': "one in which the term distinguishes a person's self as a whole (including, perhaps, his body) from other people, and the other in which it denotes a particular part of the mind characterized by special attributes and functions." Both in the depiction of the ego in the *Project* (1895) and in the description of the anatomy of the mind in *The Ego and the Id*, says Strachey, the term is used in the second sense. Yet in some of the writings Freud produced in between, "the 'ego' seems to correspond rather to the 'self'. It is not always easy, however, to draw a line between these two senses of the word" (Strachey, 1923, pp. 7–8).

Freud (1930) wrote very little about this topic. I consider more significant his claim that, normally, "there is nothing of which we are more certain than the feeling of our own self, of our own ego" (Freud, 1930, p. 65). While it is hard to conceptualize the idea, we know our self as what we always are, we might say, what we recognize about ourselves – our identity. In the above-quoted work, Stern agrees with Freud's observation.

At first, Winnicott assumed that the self was an easy concept to define. Yet having to do so in response to a request from his French translator, he confesses that as soon as he started writing about the word *self*, he realized that he was not certain about what he meant by it:

> I found I had written the following: 'For me the self, which is not the ego, is the person who is me, who has a totality based on the operation of the maturational process (...) The self finds itself naturally placed in the body, but may in certain circumstances become dissociated from the body in the eyes and facial expression of the mother and in the mirror which can come to represent the mother's face.
>
> (Winnicott, [1970] 1989, p. 271)

In the next chapter I discuss this author's concepts of true and false self.

Kohut (1977), for his part, argues that the self cannot be known in its essence. "We cannot," he says,

> by introspection and empathy, penetrate to the self per se; only its introspectively or empathically perceived manifestations are open to us (...) 'the self' is not the concept of an abstract science, but a generalization derived from empirical data (...) We can collect data concerning the way in which the set of introspectively or empathically perceived inner experiences to which we later refer as 'I' is gradually established, and we can observe certain characteristic vicissitudes of this experience.
>
> (Kohut, 1977, p. 310)

Schafer, in turn, understands that our identity is formed by several narrative selves, and agrees with Mitchell (1991) that mental health also depends on our ability to tolerate the manifold facets that constitute us.

Winnicott, Kohut, and those who inspired them (Ferenczi, Balint, Sullivan, Fairbairn, Mahler, Hartmann, and Erikson)[8]

The perspectives of the authors we are studying here are based on the ideas of thinkers who tried to explain some phenomena that have been thoroughly examined by our contemporaries. In the history of science, ideas are often formulated that do not take hold. As a case in point, Aristarchus of Samos described Heliocentrism in 270 AC, more than fifteen centuries ahead of Copernicus. Giordano Bruno and Galileo, however, paid years later for Copernicus's announcement, the former with his life and the latter by having to publicly recant his ideas – the price of advancing theories that power was unwilling to accept.

All across the history of science, power and truth have been at war. They only complemented and accepted each other when power appropriated the definition of truth in each historical period. At the same time, theory emerges from context, as Guntrip (1971) points out. This author states that "all theories, especially those about human nature, are conditioned by the cultural era, the prevailing intellectual climate, and the dominant ideas of the time in which they are developed" (Guntrip, 1971, p. 10). This is what happened in the history of psychoanalysis (why would our discipline be an exception?). Just as an example, many of the ideas that Winnicott would eventually formulate may already be found in Balint and Ferenczi's work.

This section focuses on the authors that preceded Winnicott and Kohut (without attempting to summarize their work), since I understand that they are all part of a common core; their way of looking at phenomena generated a theory that did not centre on the vicissitudes of instincts. We should recall here that these authors do not see psychic conflict as the starting point of psychic pathology but take other motivations into account. I mentioned earlier that analysts tend to talk about the early psyche as the period that goes from birth to the culmination of the Oedipus complex (the child's "pre-history"), and consider the evolution of instincts as the backbone of the definition of development. Until the appearance of the precursors I discuss next, and especially until Winnicott and Kohut set forth their ideas, there were but marginal references in the literature to the significant role played by the environment and to other motivational factors in child development.

It is worth insisting that when Winnicott states that the baby does not exist, he is referring to the impossibility to view the baby as a differentiated psychic entity. The baby is not the "owner" of its incipient psyche. I already pointed out that in the earliest stages of development, the human baby, so dependent and immature, needs objects that will hold it (materially and metaphorically), that will handle it and facilitate its integration into the object world (Winnicott), that will reflect it and allow the idealized fusion that will make it feel safe (Kohut). If these objects, embodied in the maternal figure (who is not necessarily the baby's biological mother), respond appropriately, they will be experienced as the continuity of the self, which will gradually develop.

These authors' perspective is characterized by its emphasis on the specific response of the objects that are present in the baby's environment. If the latter is unhealthy, the consequences will appear later in life. We are, then, dealing with theories that prioritize the environment in which the human creature develops, regardless of instinct evolution, as the main factor in the achievement of good health. If the environment fails (if the early bonds are inadequate to ensure development), subjects will present with deficit pathology.

While the authors considered here formulated many ideas, I only discuss those that are found in Winnicott and Kohut's work. Sandor Ferenczi (1873–1933) and the Balints were the emblematic promoters of the creative Hungarian school of psychoanalysis. Ferenczi lived until he was 60 years old and left a substantial oeuvre where he questions the psychoanalysis of his time. It is important to read the primary sources, for he is one of those authors who are often questioned as "transgressors" but are seldom read. It was not until recently (so many decades after his death!) that his work started to be reassessed.

Ferenczi was Freud's patient for a total of 90 sessions at different times. His most original works were published in the last decade of his life. One of the most creative ones, after the publication of *Talassa* (1924), is "The Elasticity of Psycho-Analytic Technique" (1928), where he develops the concept of *Einfülhung* (empathy), which Kohut will take up again.[9] Ferenczi claims that empathy will guide the therapist's attitude when deciding how and when to interpret. (We should recall here that for Kohut, empathy draws the boundaries of analysts' field of action with regard to potential knowledge about their analysands, and that outside these boundaries we are treading on uncertain grounds.)

Michel Balint, who wrote many of his papers together with his wife based on a practice with severely ill patients, addresses an array of topics. In relation to our two authors, we should point to *The Basic Fault* (1968) as his most significant work. This fault, a discernible feeling in severely ill patients, emerges due to the failure of the maternal object to respond to the child's (preverbal, pre-Oedipal) needs. Balint's discovery gave rise to what was later developed as *deficit theory* (Killingmo, 1978).

Fairbairn (1889–1964), it is worth reiterating, suggests (particularly after 1940) that the libido seeks objects rather than pleasure, that the erogenous zones are mediating channels, and that libidinal phases are "techniques of the ego" that regulate object relations. In this way, he lays the foundations for a notion that we might call "primary impulse" (the search for objects as the key driving force of the psyche). This notion differs from Freud's idea of "secondary impulses," as the latter refers to the fact that sexuality rests on self-conservation instincts (anaclisis). Sexuality becomes blurred as a psychic motivation, for it is their need for love (interest) that babies primarily aim to satisfy. Thence the complex psychic structuring suggested by Fairbairn, where we find "ego functions indissolubly linked to objects in the constitution of a psychic reality that excludes the internal world's instinctive hydraulics-mechanics" (Dupetit, 1986, no pagination).

As we indicated earlier, Fairbairn reformulates the theory of the drives; he does not see the psyche as a result of the conflict between drives and defences. Neither does he agree with the existence of a death instinct. According to this author, first there is a relationship, the object bond, and then this bond is libidinally charged. Impulses are subsidiary to the self and are not a source of energy independent of structures. Context was one of his bones of contention with Freud. Fairbairn believed that the nineteenth century was "dominated by the Helmholtzian conception that the physical universe consisted in a conglomeration of inert, immutable and indivisible particles to which motion was imparted by a fixed quantity of energy separate from the particles themselves" (Fairbairn, [1952] 2001, p. 126). If we look at the concept of libido from Fairbairn's perspective and combine it with other authors' postulates (those that point to the self as individuals' psychological core), we can see that classic metapsychology leaves an entire early bonding world out of the field of the psychoanalysis of neuroses.

In the US, Harry S. Sullivan, a psychiatrist and psychoanalyst who lived during the first half of the twentieth century (1892–1949) and devoted himself primarily to the study of schizophrenic patients, developed a theory that is as interesting as it is rarely quoted. This author's views on personality development (interpersonal theory, in his own terms), which doubtless constitute the basis for many of today's intersubjectivist ideas, were influenced by the culturalist movement (White, Sapir, Mead, Meyer, and Benedict). He argues that humans are the result of their interactions with their fellow beings since their birth (Sullivan, 1953). The most important motivations of the human psyche are attaining satisfaction and safety. The former is based on biology, while the yearning for safety is a cultural product.

Sullivan considers that humans are always part of a situation. There are no isolated human beings; we are always interacting with those around us. Based on our biological substratum, we are the result of our bonds with our fellow beings since our birth. These ideas allow Sullivan to integrate a psycho-somato-social notion of humankind. In his lectures at the William A. White Institute in 1944 and 1945, he suggested that illness is tied to interpersonal communication, as most mental disorders result from, and are perpetuated by, inadequate interactions where anxiety hinders communication processes.

Hartmann (1894–1970), for his part, develops his theoretical hypotheses based on old positivist biological models, and from there he postulates the existence of a conflict-free sphere in the ego. The maturation of the ego, according to this author, results from the reciprocal, uninterrupted interaction between the body's needs and environmental influences (Fenichel, 1945). He sees psychoanalysis as a general psychology, and is interested in mental functions such as memory and knowledge and, in particular, in defensive systems (Bleichmar and Bleichmar, 1989). The transference repeats only Oedipal drive features of patients' history, and hence the earlier stages are not accessible. Those elements tied to the actual person of the analyst acquire great significance because it is with them that the rational, conflict-free aspects of the patient establish a relationship, and they facilitate the appearance of the therapeutic alliance. From these ideas derive the concepts developed by authors such as Rapaport, Zetzel, and Greenson.

Erik Erikson (1902–1994) played a prominent role in North American psychoanalysis. This author discussed individuals' potential for development at every stage of their lives, and conceived the notion of life cycle. The life cycle is divided into eight stages and does not end in adolescence, as could be concluded from Freud's ideas concerning the Oedipus complex. Rather, it encompasses the entire adult life and old age. If the main issues appearing in each stage are adequately solved, individuals can healthily move on to the next stage. These issues are:

Trust vs. Mistrust
Autonomy vs. Shame
Initiative vs. Guilt
Industry vs. Inferiority
Identity vs. Role Confusion
Intimacy vs. Isolation
Generativity vs. Stagnation
Ego Integrity vs. Despair

The first five correspond to childhood and early adolescence, and the other three, to adulthood and old age. Each stage has its own specific emotional crises, which are affected and determined by both biology and culture. In each we may find a healthy or unhealthy development. If we look at the first stage, we see that, in agreement with Winnicott and Kohut's ideas, the baby's gradual acquisition of this trusting attitude will depend on the surrounding objects' healthy response to its primitive needs, a response that will be influenced by society's upbringing requirements.

Erikson ([1982] 1997) illustrates this complex operation with a description of the Sioux's childrearing methods, and stresses that babies will perfect their adaptive functions based on the most trivial everyday habits. The Sioux mothers were attentive and generous toward their babies, but during breastfeeding and during the teething period, they would "playfully aggravate the infant boy's ready rage in such a way that the greatest possible degree of latent ferocity was provoked." The author adds:

> This was apparently to be channelized later into customary play and then into work, hunting and warring demanding competent aggressiveness against prey and enemy. Thus, we concluded, primitive cultures, beyond giving specific meanings to early bodily and interpersonal experience in order to create the 'right' emphases on both organ modes and social modalities, appear to channelize carefully and systematically the energies thus provoked and deflected; and they give consistent supernatural meaning to the infantile anxieties that they have exploited by such provocation.
>
> (Erikson, [1982] 1997, p. 35)

Erikson's contribution to the theories of self school authors is highly significant, especially regarding epigenetic development and adaptation, for it takes into account the social requirements embodied in childrearing actions.

As to Margaret Mahler (1968, 1975), based on numerous observations of babies and their mothers in the 1960s and 1970s, she explains empirical phenomena while taking into consideration both the Freudian and the ego psychology models and relating them to Fairbairn's ideas about object relations. She proposes three phases of normal development: a first autistic phase that lasts four weeks and corresponds to an absolute primary narcissism, when the baby remains isolated and immersed in itself; a symbiotic phase of unity with the mother that lasts approximately until the sixth month; and a third phase of separation-individuation that comprises four sub-phases (differentiation, practicing, rapprochement, and object constancy). Individuality is then consolidated, and the baby achieves integration and an acceptably stable object constancy (between two and three years of age).

Separation is considered an intrapsychic achievement, while individuation starts with the awareness of one's own being. Mahler believes that in child psychosis the symbiotic relationship is either absent or severely distorted, while in the autistic syndrome the child cannot use its mother to face stimuli whose origin is as yet uncertain and that threaten the child as an individual entity. The autistic defence is an extreme attempt to hallucinate negatively the existence of the world of living objects (Dio de Bleichmar, 1977). Difficulties may emerge in each phase that will translate into a later pathology, which may be autistic or symbiotic.

It is impossible to summarize all the other authors who influenced the work of Winnicott and Kohut, but I cannot fail to mention Bowlby (1907–1990), whose work I discuss later.

Notes

1　This chapter and some of the following ones are based on lectures developed for APdeBA's remote courses between 2004 and 2013.
2　Perspective is always a product of the existing social imaginary at a certain historical moment. The value of art – and psychoanalysis has certainly much of the arts in its mode of operation! – lies in that it facilitates the development of a hitherto unappreciated point of view, thus enabling us to find new formulations concerning our observations. Ultimately, such development will lead to the creation of new facts. Thus, Alberti stated that he could finally see the world as God had created it when he came into contact with Renaissance perspective, inaugurated by Brunelleschi (Berger, 1963), and five centuries later Dali claimed, "When I see, I invent" (Ades, 1982, p. 64).
3　We can hypothesize that these ideas were too advanced for their time, when analysts were required to remain faithful to the Freudian approach, if not to Freud's figure. Moreover, these innovators probably were unable or did not know how to gain the political power that would have facilitated the dissemination of their ideas.
4　We should recall here the first words of the *Project*, which Freud writes in 1895 and quickly shelves:

> The intention of this project is to furnish us with a psychology which shall be a natural science: its aim, that is, is to represent psychical processes as quantitatively determined states of specifiable material particles and so to make them plain and void of contradictions.
>
> (Freud, 1950a [1895], p. 283).

5　Blending epochs and objects of study, and as an example, we can consider Stern's (1985) viewpoint:

> Much evidence about the feeding patterns of existing primitive societies (...) suggest that throughout most history babies were fed very frequently, on the slightest demand – as often as twice an hour. Since most infants were carried about with the mother, against her body, she would sense the infant getting even slightly restless and would initiate short and frequent feedings, maybe just a few sips to keep the level of activations low.
>
> (Stern, 1985, p. 237)

The corollary of this analysis is that the breastfeeding drama we witness today is a product of our system, which creates great stimulation and activation in the shape of hunger, followed by an abrupt fall. Satiation becomes a phenomenon of equal intensity and drama as hunger but with an opposite direction.
6　Nietzsche (1972) says with his tremendous voice:

> The strength of conceptions does not, therefore, depend on their degree of truth, but on their antiquity, their embodiment, their character as conditions of life. Where life and knowledge seemed to conflict, there has never been serious contention; denial and doubt have there been regarded as madness.
>
> (Nietzsche, 2006 [1910], p. 83)

7　It is worth stressing once again that psychopathology depends on a certain frame of reference, which, in turn, is a product of the current culture. Psychopathology usually evolves "on the edges" of classification categories. For example, borderline disorders appear on the border between psychosis and neurosis, but they will soon have to be distinguished from schizoid personalities. The latter, in turn, will have to be differentiated from ambulatory schizophrenias and severe neuroses. Our "new ways of seeing" make our taxonomy increasingly complex.

8 Laplanche and Pontalis (1971) discuss erotogenic zones. From the perspective of libidinal development, they state that we must give consideration to the fact that "these zones, at the beginnings of psychosexual development, constitute the favoured paths of exchange with the surroundings, while at the same time soliciting the most attention, care – and consequently stimulation – from the mother" (Laplanche and Pontalis, 1973, p. 155).

9 Published in English in *Final Contributions to the Problems and Methods of Psychoanalysis*, edited by Michael Balint, New York: Brunner/Mazel, pp. 87–102. (T. N.).

2   Early psychic development in the work of Winnicott and Kohut

Some biographical information on Donald W. Winnicott

Donald W. Winnicott was born in 1896 in Plymouth, England. He was the youngest of three children; his sisters were five and seven years older. He started medical school at Cambridge University when he was 18 years old but was forced to drop out with the outbreak of World War I. He became a navy surgeon, and was able to finish his studies in London in 1920. It was at this time that he came into contact with Freud's work. Some years later he started his first analysis with James Strachey and was admitted to the British Psycho-Analytical Society. He was also a paediatrician, and kept practicing until a few years before this death.

In 1923 he started working at the Paddington Green Children's Hospital in London. When Klein settled in London, he began supervision with her, and after finishing his analysis with Strachey, he had further analysis with Joan Riviere. His position in the British society, equidistant with Klein's and with that of the newly arrived Anna Freud, situated him as the leading figure of the middle group (there were three groups, namely, Anna Freud's, Melanie Klein's, and the numerous middle group). This group sought to integrate A. Freud and Klein's ideas and build on them. Balint, Bowlby, Khan, Rycroft, Milner, and Klauber were some of its members. Winnicott presided the British Psycho-Analytical Society for two terms, 1956–1959 and 1965–1968. He remarried to the psychiatric social worker Clare Britton, his collaborator, during World War II, and died without offspring in 1971.

The early psyche

Winnicott worked with children, adolescents, and adults throughout his professional life, and recorded hundreds of cases. His patients presented with a very broad range of illnesses – from neurosis to borderline personality, asocial psychopathy, psychosis, and perversion. His writing style is also relevant, for it is consistent with his nature and his way of thinking. Kahn says about him that he talked about things that were "so patently clear but rarely spoken of" (Khan and Masud, 1958, p. xii). Perhaps in Winnicott's work more than in any one else's, his style, both playful and deep, mirrors the theories he formulates, in particular, his concept of play and of human modes of communication (a direct, explicit form of communication, and an indirect one that would lose meaning were it fully explicit).

For this author, babies are born with inherited potentials that will unfold depending on their encounters with the first objects in the environment. It is a vitalist approach (Ferrater Mora, 1984), doubtlessly influenced by Heidegger's existentialism as well as by Buber and Bergson. Today we would consider him a hermeneutist insofar as he sees the object as immersed in a relationship and shares Gadamer and Ricoeur's views that interpretation facilitates our understanding of events. Such position takes into account people's history and clearly differs from structuralist approaches.

The environment facilitates development, which is promoted by babies' inherited potential. It is thanks to the baby's encounter with the environment that its spontaneous gesture can emerge and grow as an expression of its creativity. This is the paradigm that governs Winnicott's original oeuvre from beginning ("Primitive Emotional Development" in 1945) to end. Baby and environment constitute an initial unit, thence Winnicott's assertion that the baby does not exist as an entity. He is alluding to its inextricable link to the maternal object, which will enable the development of inherited potentials on the slow path toward independence. The failure of the indispensable object will interrupt the baby's existential continuity. Such continuity is key to this author's idea of psychic health, and its interruption is defined as traumatic. Continuity involves movement, progressively being, becoming. Winnicott coined the expression "going-on-being," using the present participle, a verbal form that signals progression.[1]

Babies need their objects to integrate, to live in their body (personalization), and to make contact with reality (realization). Faced with the baby's needs, it is the maternal object that performs the roles of holding, handling, and object-presenting. We should note here that we are talking about needs rather than sexual desires. In *Playing and Reality* Winnicott states as follows:

> it is not instinctual satisfaction that makes a baby begin to be, to feel that life is real, to find life worth living. In fact, instinctual gratifications start off as part-functions and they become *seductions* unless based on a well-established capacity in the individual person for total experience, and for experience in the area of transitional phenomena. It is the self that must precede the self's use of instinct; the rider must ride the horse, not be run away with.
>
> (Winnicott, [1971] 1989, pp. 98–99; author's emphasis)

Especially at the very beginning, the self's needs (continuity, intimacy, mutuality) are constantly there, whereas instincts only assail the baby periodically. If it can meet the self's needs, the baby will be able to incorporate instinctual demands in a natural way.

Winnicott will call the maternal function that satisfies elementary needs, which is configured from the baby's point of view, "environment-mother," and the maternal function that satisfies instinct needs, "object-mother." Children embark on a journey that goes from absolute dependence to independence, passing through relative dependence. If everything goes well, says Winnicott, they achieve self and object integration, personalization, and the beginning of a relationship with the other. These achievements are made possible by the mother's holding, handling, and reality-presenting functions.

This "good enough" mother (good because she is simply enough and not too much, an achievement that does not require special skills) is usually sensitive, vulnerable, and resilient, but also knows about her hatred, which she does not negate (hatred tied to her baby's dependence and the responsibility demanded by her position). She also wishes to be eaten by her baby. These maternal features develop while she is in a state of preoccupation for her baby (a functional schizoid maternal state preceding the birth of the child that persists for a few months) that Winnicott calls Primary Maternal Preoccupation.

Proper environmental responses will allow the baby to feel the omnipotence of having created the object according to its own needs. (Just as that primitive pleasure ego described by Freud, this Winnicottian baby might say, "The breast is part of me" and "Just as I create it, so I destroy it.") Such belief, made possible by the maternal function, rapidly becomes less absolute (with the transition process and the incorporation of other objects from reality, absolute omnipotence will become omnipotence with regard to handling objects).

These vicissitudes put the baby in contact with its ability to create, and the experience of creation is essential to the development of the self. Babies will be able to feel authentic and develop their own original ideas, and thereby "be" and settle in their own body. They also experience the paradoxical feeling of having invented their own objects. We are at the beginning, when the object is still "subjective," that is, created – and destroyed – by the baby, who makes the object appear when it needs it and disappear when it does not want to have anything to do with it. The baby loves the object cruelly and destroys it at will in order to give life to it anew. In this primitive love we recognize the origin of aggression, which, according to Winnicott, is unintentional during this stage.

Next will come a logical, and not necessarily chronological, sequence tied to the transitional stage. During this stage, (transitional) objects acquire a material reality that makes ownership possible (first not-me possession). Possessing the object enables the baby to differentiate the self from its surroundings in a dialectical movement. Through playing, an expression of creativity rather than a product of the instincts, babies can display these new acquisitions in their connection with the real world. Symbol formation goes hand in hand with the gradual separation from the first maternal object. It is here, in this second stage, that children's cultural life begins.

Gradually, the environment-mother and the object-mother are integrated, and concern arises as a new feeling (from approximately eight months on). The first depressive feelings appear, corresponding to Klein's depressive position. At this time, babies perceive their primitive, unintentional aggression against the objects around them, which have already become not-me, and hence feel responsible for this aggression. They start feeling guilt and attempting to repair.

The mother must survive the baby's hatred (aggression) at different times. Based on these early experiences, the baby will be able to dream and create fantasies. If the mother repeatedly fails to respond to such hatred, the baby will repress it or will continue to feel omnipotent, which is the basis of severe obsessional neuroses or antisocial behaviour.

Winnicott does not adhere to the Freudian hypothesis of a death drive. He adopts a vitalist perspective, and thus rejects any form of reduction of the organic to the inorganic. Life, in this sense, is "vital force," independent of physical-chemical phenomena. Painceira (1997) has expressed it accurately: "There is no room for the death instinct in Winnicott's thought. Life is not the expression of an instinct but of a vital impulse very close to Bergson's *élan vital*" (Painceira, 1997, p. 97). I will take up these topics again in subsequent chapters.

Early psychic development in Kohut's work

Some biographical information about Heinz Kohut

Kohut was born in 1913 in the Austrian Alps, and finished his medical studies in Vienna, where he started analysis with a friend of Freud's, August Eichorn. Shortly after Freud's forced migration to London, Kohut moved to the US to escape Nazism. He specialized in neurology in Chicago and had further analysis with Ruth Eissler. It was there that he started his training in psychiatry and psychoanalysis. In 1944 he was admitted to the Psychoanalytic Institute, where he taught Freudian theory and became a training analyst.

Paraphrasing Guntrip's words about Freud, we could say that Kohut laid the cornerstone of a new building, the "self" school, which is still under construction. His work has outlived him for two reasons. He suggested new approaches that are very valuable to contemporary psychoanalytic practice, and he trained proficient disciples who researched into their teacher's work and recreated it, while simultaneously debating with him. Thus, they expanded this work beyond the pathologies to which he had devoted his clinical practice (especially narcissistic personality disorders). Kohut was president of the North American Psychoanalytic Association (1964–1965), vice president of the International Psychoanalytical Association (1965–1973), vice president of the Sigmund Freud Archives (1971–1981), and member of the Austrian Academy of Sciences. What follows is a brief summary of his work.

a   In his writings prior to 1965, Freudian theory constitutes Kohut's frame
     of reference. He also quotes his local predecessors and contemporar-
     ies (Hartmann, Erikson, Mahler, Kris, Lowenstein), and gradually in-
     corporates original ideas – his concept of the evolution of narcissism.
     The singularity of his approach starts becoming clear in 1959 in a pa-
     per where he highlights what he views as the essential tools of analytic
     practice, namely, empathy and introspection. I am referring to "Intro-
     spection, Empathy, and Psychoanalysis: An Examination of the Rela-
     tionship Between Mode of Observation and Theory."

b   In 1966 he gives a paper in Buenos Aires where he outlines the four
     mature transformations of narcissism: empathy, humour, wisdom, and
     acceptance of the finitude of life. This article was published in *Psi-
     coanálisis de las Américas* (Paidós, 1968). The already classic papers
     "Forms and Transformations of Narcissism" (1966) and "Thoughts on
     Narcissism and Narcissistic Rage" (1972) are also from this period. Dur-
     ing this stage he systematizes the first two types of narcissistic transfer-
     ence identified in his research, which he calls *mirror transference* and
     idealizing transference.

c   In 1971 he publishes his first book, *The Analysis of the Self* (Interna-
     tional Universities Press). There he describes narcissism as a source
     of development independent of the libido, whose evolution he sees as
     biaxial – an object libido and a narcissistic libido. This conception dif-
     fers from the one that views narcissism as subordinate to object love.

d   The year 1977 marks the appearance of his second book, *The Resto-
     ration of the Self* (International Universities Press). In it, he offers an
     original description of turn-of-the-century Vienna, where psychoanal-
     ysis was born (of the social values that were favoured at the time), and
     discusses his concept of the self as containing a psyche that is the prod-
     uct of the relationship between the individual and the environment. It
     is here that Kohut radically departs from the classic theory of instincts
     and defences (conflict theory) and grounds his view in a conception that
     will eventually configure a unique line of work, the Self Psychology
     School.

e   In 1984 his last book, *How Does Analysis Cure?* (University of Chicago
     Press), comes out, which he wrote in 1981, shortly before his death. In
     1982 *The International Journal of Psychoanalysis* had published his post-
     humous essay, "Introspection, Empathy, and the Semi-Circle of Mental
     Health." This essay counters the Oedipal myth (which serves as the ba-
     sis for Freud's conflict theory) with the myth of Odysseus in order to
     justify Kohut's most elaborate ideas, based on a reparatory narcissism,
     as I pointed out earlier. This myth, rather than Oedipal rivalry, provides
     a model for the caring and protection of children – in particular, for
     intergenerational cooperation. As I discussed above, Kohut considers
     that the pathological resolution of the Oedipus complex results from the
     early abandonment of the child, from the suffering of an immature self

that is incapable of controlling its instincts. He thus distinguishes this pathological evolution (with consequences for the subject's psychopathology) from the normal Oedipal stage.

Kohut's concept of early psyche

Kohut is one of the authors who see the human environment as indispensable for the creation of the psychic structure. He tells us that the baby needs the presence of the earliest objects, its caregivers. He would certainly agree with Balint's view that these first objects are as necessary as air is to breathe. Without the basic contribution of the infant's surroundings, psychic growth is impossible. These early objects will be part of a specific environment that will promote development, thanks to their empathic connection with the subject. By way of their presence and action, they perform various complementary functions that fulfil the baby's needs; they mirror the incipient self, they are available for idealization, and later they can be signified by the subject as alter egos.

The structure of the self progressively forms in this relational matrix with early objects, which Kohut calls selfobjects (SOs). After repeated optimal responses, these objects are internalized and configure the infant's nuclear self. Over time, the infant's experiences with them will make it possible for the need for their functional presence to be less pressing. When does the internalization process start? When the selfobject gradually and adequately fails to perform its function (optimal failure) – when it ceases to be so necessary. Kohut calls this operation *transmuting internalization* (TI). SOs are cathected with the infant's narcissistic charges, which Kohut distinguishes from object charges in that the baby cannot differentiate its incipient self from the object (the SO is as part of the baby as its own hand).

Kohut describes two types of SOs for the initial stage, which mirror the child and thus confirm its innate feeling of vigour, grandeur, and perfection. They are called Mirroring Objects and are related to ambition, as we shall see later. The other objects are the ones the child admires and with which it blends, thus acquiring a feeling of calm, infallibility, and omnipotence. They are called Idealized Parental Imago. If internalized, they will be linked to the child's ideals.

The constitution of the self is a gradual process that encompasses the first life stages. TI allows the child a greater autonomy from its SOs and develops in two logical and chronological steps: (a) the experience of satisfaction with the corresponding SO; (b) the object's optimal failure (frustration that the child can tolerate because it happens at the right moment and time). The TI will enable the formation of the first structures in the self, and these structures will enable the infant to feel recognized, valued, and trusted. Kohut argues that during the second year of life, this Nuclear Self consolidates as an independent centre of initiative, integrating basic ambitions and ideals with bodily and psychic experiences that constitute a temporal and spatial unit.

As I already pointed out, for Kohut, the self is unknowable in its essence; it can only be inferred through its manifestations, and can be accessed by way of empathy and introspection. The metapsychological configuration of the self contemplates two structures, namely, the Pole of Ideals (in relation to being) and the Pole of Ambitions (in relation to having), among which a tension arc will develop. The first pole is constituted based on a relationship with an Idealized Object, a relationship that leads to the internalization of the Idealized Parental Imago. If the latter is deficient, subjects will need the object to blend with it and achieve calm and a sense of infallibility. The Pole of Ambitions, in turn, results from the union with the Mirroring Object, from which the baby will receive confirmation, approval, vigour, and grandeur.

Between the two poles, an arc of tension is established that activates the Talents and Skills with which the child can operate in life. Kohut calls it an arc of tension because it involves the "abiding flow of actual psychological activity that establishes itself between the two poles of the self, i.e., a person's basic pursuit toward which he is 'driven' by his ambitions and 'led' by his ideals" (Kohut, 1977, p. 100).[2] If these stages follow one another without traumatic interruptions, the self will be cohesive, full of life, and harmonious. Pathology, by contrast, may transform cohesion into fragmentation, suck out the life of the self, or create hypertrophy at one of the poles.

Kohut's major contributions to psychoanalysis

- We should reiterate here that Kohut combatted the prejudice that viewed narcissism as primitive and object relations as more evolved. The consequence of such prejudice was to assume that maturity (or the cure) depended on the transformation of narcissism into object libido. As an alternative, Kohut propounds two independent lines of development, neither of which is better than the other. These are the path of narcissism, and the path of instincts-objects.
- The notion of self is not an abstract idea; rather, it is always close to experience.
- The intimate proximity that facilitates understanding is established by way of empathy, which delimits the scope of psychoanalytic practice.
- Narcissism is characterized by its unique way of experiencing the object as part of the self. This bonding mode is in direct connection with the appearance of self-esteem disorders (which are not a result of the drive-defense conflict).
- Based on individuals' Narcissistic Transferences, Kohut describes Narcissistic Personality and Behaviour Disorders. The narcissistic transference will later be called "object transference of the self." The object involved will be defined as the one that is narcissistically charged, with which subjects relate in three ways: as a mirror, as an idealized figure, and as an alter ego. These bonds are indispensable for survival and

development, as the child needs to be mirrored and will seek a figure (a selfobject) it can idealize and, later on, an object that will function as a peer (alter ego). The presence of the narcissistic transference mode in the analysis will depend on the deficits of the selfobjects that interacted with the subject in the past. Such deficits will result in an arrested development that may resume its course if the analyst responds empathically in the manner of the needed selfobject.

Summing up, then, for Kohut, subjects have a "transference capital" that has two origins: (a) deficits caused by the lack of availability or empathy of primary objects, which should have met the baby's basic needs; and (b) Oedipal conflicts. Like Winnicott, Kohut rejects the death drive hypothesis. The narcissistic pathologies he describes are Primary Disorders (psychoses, borderline personalities, addictions) and Secondary Disorders (NPD, neuroses) of the self.

* Psychic development is ongoing. It does not end in an "apparatus" that processes drives (which are discharged or sublimated and are in conflict with repression) and whose purpose is the constitution of the superego or maturation through genitality. Kohut points out that Freud was concerned with characterizing the Guilty Man, driven by instincts and defending himself from them, and that his paradigm was the Oedipus complex (based on the intergenerational struggle). The latter served as a model for conflict and represented the core of psychic development. Kohut considers that this viewpoint universalizes conflict and is restricted to the psychobiological realm. He advances a different paradigm based on what he calls Tragic Man, who searches for his destiny with his father's support (intergenerational cooperation).

Kohut substitutes Odysseus for Oedipus, and argues that this new approach is psychological and detached from instinct determinism. He claims that we must distinguish between the Oedipal phase or stage and the pathological evolution of that phase, that is, the Oedipus complex. If development is possible, thanks to a proper articulation with the environment, the child will undergo the normal Oedipal "period or stage," where intergenerational cooperation will prevail over competition and hatred. The boy and his father will feel pride for each other and will not wish the other's death.

* Kohut also contributed to the study of the context in which psychoanalysis develops in each period (see epigraph to Chapter 1). Based on the observation of the current social environment and the set of values that prevailed when psychoanalysis was born (knowledge and independence), he suggests that the values that are cherished but scarce today are the need for the presence of a fellow being, understanding, and object availability.

Notes

1 Winnicott uses the present participle as a noun to emphasize the continuity of the action, the constant motion, the continuity of being, and the process of becoming, which are paradigmatic concepts in his theory. As Pontalis (1971) asserts, the words fantasying, dreaming, living, and holding suggest movement, something that is in the process of happening rather than a finished product.

2 Lerner and I (Lerner and Nemirovsky, 1989a) consider that empathy may be defined in three different ways. First, as a phenomenon that is inherent in human communication. In our relationship with the other, we reconstruct inside ourselves, in an isomorphic manner, his or her psychic states. To this end, we have developed certain implicit notions of human behaviour and emotional states. When analysts understand empathically, an experiential resonance has taken place inside them that is isomorphic with that of the patient. Second, we can think of it as a way of acquiring knowledge. It is a spontaneous phenomenon that happens beyond the observer's control. Nonetheless, this does not mean that it is a single act; rather, it is a process that leads to knowledge. To acquire this knowledge, we resort to mechanisms such as imitation, imagination, evocation, and momentary, partial and controlled identification. Finally, empathy may be viewed as a therapeutic tool, as it facilitates the creation of a therapeutic field of interaction in which the analytic dialogue may unfold. Transference is thus made possible. Empathy is a suitable instrument to enable personalization (the integration, cohesion, and consolidation of the self) in patients who suffer disorders originating in empathetic failure with their early objects. In sum, I believe that it would be possible to reconstruct a situation involving someone else by way of intellectual or conceptual approaches, but the potential for success is minimal if empathetic resonance does not take place.

3 Similarities and differences between Winnicott and Kohut's approaches[1]

This chapter discusses contributions by Kohut and Winnicott that represented a significant departure from current psychoanalytic thought. These authors' ideas did not merely broaden Freudian theory and practice; they were complex notions that made up actual theoretical frameworks and continued to develop through debate and controversy. I believe that three significant factors were instrumental in the appearance of these new perspectives: (a) changes in subjectivity tied to a new sociohistorical juncture; (b) the application of the psychoanalytic method to the treatment of children and families; and (c) greater experience with borderline and psychotic patients. Changes in the social imaginary and the considerable growth of the empirical basis, as well as, most likely, their identification with Freud's daring traits as a researcher (an identification that did not imply blindly following in his steps), led these two paradigmatic authors to rethink numerous issues associated with our discipline's basic theoretical concepts. These range from the motivation behind psychic acts to psychoanalytic technique.

Elsewhere (Nemirovsky, 1993) I point out that only by forcing our reading of Freud's treatment protocols could we find a recurring and invariable psychoanalytic method. These cases do not show a "classic" way of addressing psychic suffering. Freud's approach involves inquiring into the vicissitudes of his clinical practice, developing his theory based on that practice, and going back to his patients with a different perspective in an ongoing cycle where identifying a beginning and an end would be arbitrary. The way he conceptualizes his practice is also atypical, for his endlessly shifting oeuvre hinders any attempt to fix concepts through working definitions. His central ideas, linked to the early notion of psychoanalysis, configure a metapsychology that allows different readings. These readings, in turn, open different paths that constitute the foundations of the various schools of thought making up present-day psychoanalysis. Perhaps we say "classic" out of a wish to find reassuring, indisputable knowledge.

These are some of the reasons behind the need to form schools, inherent in our discipline so far. Therefore, when dealing with analysts who have similar outlooks, I believe it is appropriate to ask what would be the common denominator. What should be a necessary part of analytic training? What brings analysts together? What makes us consider ourselves part of the same "species"? The answer to these questions is elusive. How far we are from, and how reassured we would feel by, having such a categorical definition as the one provided by Freud in his efforts to consolidate the Psychoanalytic Movement in 1922! He outlines the following as the pillars of the discipline:

> The assumption that there are unconscious processes, the recognition of the theory of resistance and repression, the appreciation of the importance of sexuality and of the Oedipus complex – these constitute the principal subject-matter of psychoanalysis and the formulations of its theory. No one who cannot accept them all should count himself a psychoanalyst.
>
> (Freud, 1923A, p. 247)

I also acknowledge our Freudian paternity. We probably share the notion of unconscious (the descriptive rather than the systematic notion) and its staging through the transference. We also have in common the ethical attitude derived from the analyst's position and the search for truth (focusing on the path, the search itself). Nevertheless, we know very well that when a scientist of Freud's stature offers such a precise text, populated by requirements of belonging and, therefore, by exclusions, it is because he is adopting a political-institutional perspective and is more concerned with the establishment of a peer group, a psychoanalytic movement than with discussing psychoanalytic concepts.

If we attempted to find a totalizing and precise definition of psychoanalysis today, it would be impossible to narrow it down. Do we come together through ideas, perspectives, and the vertex from where we look at clinical practice? Or perhaps through the analytic attitude, the position of the analyst in his or her work?[2] Is the idea of ethics univocal and hence the common denominator for analysts from different schools? Simplifying, it is obviously the acceptance of the existence of the unconscious that brings us together. Yet I consider that it is especially our position in relation to our ordinary actions with our patients that defines most of us as analysts.

It is unlikely that contemporary analysts would accept all the requirements demanded by Freud's 1922 categorical imperative. Moreover, to define a sense of belonging, we would focus on the two issues I mentioned previously – the obvious recognition of unconscious processes and the practitioner's position in relation to the patient. These are not very precise requirements. For now, however, they are as insufficient as they are necessary, and are likely to appeal to the greatest number of analysts. At the same time, pointing to the notions of resistance and repression as essential components would cause endless debate.

It would be impossible to agree upon how to include topics such as patient resistance/analyst resistance and narcissistic resistance/repression/dissociation. Regarding the other elements in Freud's statement, that is, sexuality and the Oedipus complex, they would not be rejected by anyone, but there would probably be some disagreement about their place in the definition of psychoanalysis. Not every colleague would ascribe them a key status or consider them a major motivation for psychic development. We could wonder, for instance, if we should also incorporate Narcissus along with Oedipus, or even neosexualities, not to mention attachment theories.[3]

To the extent that psychoanalysis is a cultural product, theory, technique, and the concept of psychopathology are constantly evolving, and hence diagnoses evolve as well. These changes reflect the ways in which our social organization and customs shape mental pathology. The focus on the environment has led me to revisit psychoanalytic frames of reference that view the relationship with the objects that are present in the environment, and not only the drives and their vicissitudes, as critical to human development, and these objects' absence, failure, or inadequate functioning as a major factor in the aetiology of mental illness. In this sense, H. Bleichmar's (1997) contribution is significant. This author suggests that the psyche is a structure composed of

> multiple motivational systems or modules that, in their interplay, set psychic activity in motion or tend to block it (...) These systems mobilize different types of desires – of self-preservation, sexual, narcissistic, aggressive, and so on – (...) that establish different modes of intrapsychic or intersubjective defences.
>
> (Bleichmar, 1997, p. 20)

Quoting Laplanche, Bleichmar recalls that when he abandoned the seduction theory, Freud pointed to endogenous drives as the main aetiological factor, without attaching any significance to the role of the other in the very constitution of the drives. Precisely, the "decentering of the drive" is an important point of convergence of Winnicott and Kohut's basic ideas.[4] My goal is to discuss their main contributions to psychoanalysis (as well as some of their similarities and differences) in terms of their usefulness to understand problems that are increasingly present in our consulting rooms. However, I do not intend to analyse these contributions systematically.

Historical concepts, recent concepts

> The order that our mind imagines is like a net, or like a ladder, built to attain something. But afterwards you must throw the ladder away, because you discover that, even if it was useful, it was meaningless.
>
> Umberto Eco, *The Name of the Rose*, p. 142

I already quoted Freud's definition of psychoanalysis from 1922. Many years later, and after the expansion of the discipline, we could hardly agree with him unless we added concepts and clarifications. Today we would not be likely to accept a single definition or, perhaps, we should not insist on finding one; by pursuing the advantages of unification, we run the risk of reducing valuable notions. We will only be able to identify, as I did earlier, shared elements that define our work and distinguish us from other therapists. We will find that infantile sexuality, transference, and repression are not univocal terms. Moreover, we would add other paradigmatic concepts. Perhaps we would redefine ideas that were only marginally considered by Freud, for instance, psychotic and narcissistic transferences, countertransference, and so on. Furthermore, we should discuss the idea of sexuality (restricted or expanded; primary, or secondary to certain needs) and the hitherto central Oedipus complex: Do we talk about an early or a late complex? Or, should we incorporate Kohut's suggestion of an "Oedipal phase" in the developmental process that the self will undergo almost without conflict when everything goes well?

By way of clinical work and the metapsychological constructions on psychic life offered by each original author, we arrive at the question of motivation – what it is that sets the psyche in motion so that it can travel through the path of complexity. Discerning the motivations of psychic life, which drive its existence, will allow us, perhaps, to understand and encompass pathological phenomena derived from their disruption. In this sense, we should recall, once again, the four basic origins of psychic pathology posited by Bleichmar (1997):

a   the classic one, conflict;
b   the failure of the external object, that is, its inability to contribute to satisfying basic human developmental needs;
c   trauma, which occurs when the object is persecuted, terrorized, accused, or controlled in an abusive way; and
d   the original pathological inscription, that is, when the subject identifies with the parents' pathology.

In this way, not only do we take into account the Oedipal conflict (sexual desire as the driving force of the psyche), as does the first version of psychoanalysis, but also incorporate other driving forces that interrelate and form a complex weave. Moreover, if we work within an interdisciplinary framework, we can rethink psychoanalysis from the perspective of neuroscience.[5] From this perspective, we could review all forms of psychopathology, among them, hypochondriac disorders, certain forms of depression, anxiety disorders, borderline personalities, and organ neuroses, all clinical pictures for which no organic lesions could be detected in the past. Today, thanks to neuroscientific developments and new brain imaging techniques, we may be able to find an organic component, and this is even more likely in the case of psychoses.

In view of the complexity of the various scientific developments within and without the field of psychoanalysis, it would seem that the definitions of basic psychoanalytic notions are not broad enough or could be challenged from a variety of angles. I believe that rather than to define our paradigms from different theoretical perspectives, we need (and quite urgently) to find concepts that encompass the new clinical phenomena we are seeing in our consulting rooms and to incorporate the progress made inside, outside, and on the borders of our discipline. In frequent conversations with colleagues, we have wondered what theoretical concepts we could use to explain phenomena as ineffable (and as common today) as those brought by our patients, who, half baffled, half distressed, tell us they feel "numb," "unreal," "empty," "fragile," "non-existent," or "transparent."

It will not be easy to find an explanatory tool, a broad-enough metapsychology that will not deprive clinical phenomena from their richness, that will not squeeze the facts observed into a narrow mould.[6] Lipovetsky, social observer and lucid essayist, claims that "Don Juan is dead; a new, much more disturbing figure rises, Narcissus, enslaved by himself in his crystal dome" (Lipovetsky, 1986, pp. 32–33). And he adds later:

> Patients no longer suffer distinctive symptoms, but rather vague, blurred disorders; mental pathology abides by the law of the times, which tends to reduce rigidities and dissolve stable relevance. Neurotic tension has been replaced by narcissistic lightness. An inability to feel, an emotional void – desubstantiation – has reached its end, revealing the truth of the narcissistic process as a strategy of the void.
>
> (ibid., pp. 77–78)

McDougall (1980) is probably taking this social perspective into account when she argues that rather than with desire, the search for the other is connected with the psychic economy of needs. It is this psychic economy that serves as a foundation for addictive behaviour and perverse organizations of sexuality. In these organizations, sexuality becomes a drug. This author agrees with Green, who claims that today's psychoanalytic myth is Hamlet, not Oedipus.[7] Green also argues as follows:

> I believed that what had changed since Freud was probably less the population of analysands than the analysts' way of listening to them. Certainly one must not rule out the fact that one encounters fewer neurotics than in Freud's day, if only for the reason that this population is more diluted because of the greater number of analysts. But above all, it was the year of the analyst that was no longer the same. Nowadays one's hearing is more sensitive to picking up conflicts that are laden with archaic potential, which perhaps passed unnoticed in the past.
>
> (Green, 2001, p. 11)

I wonder if these contributions, based on paradigms that attach great significance to social factors (such as those suggested by observers of cultural movements), can meet our need to find comprehensive, integrating metapsychologies that will enable us to understand complex clinical phenomena. Taking these difficulties into account, we can infer that one of the features that render our profession impossible is that when we reach an acceptable level of knowledge about the pathology we must tackle, changes occur both in our object of study and in our clinical work, and therefore in our theories.[8] At least, however, we are learning that we must open our field to other disciplines and engage in a productive dialogue with the sciences of culture and with the neurosciences.

Some of Winnicott and Kohut's contributions

Clinical practice with complex patients led me to Winnicott and Kohut's writings, and continued work with these patients increased my adherence to these thinkers' approaches. Their thoughts are always tied to their interaction with patients. Even when these thoughts are formulated at a conceptual, abstract level, they remain close to empirical facts and are, therefore, useful while opening new paths.[9] The pathologies studied by both authors develop amid failed encounters and bonding disorders. They emerge at a historical time when human beings' psychological suffering is the result of their way of life and of social relations, about which so much has been said by students of post-industrial society. Let us look at some similarities and differences between Winnicott and Kohut.[10]

Similarities

While both acknowledge Freudian theory as their foundation, their conceptions are not focused on the vicissitudes of sexuality or on instinctual determinism. Rather, the centre of attention (the basic object of study, the minimum expression) is always the bond. They attach great significance to environmental factors in human childrearing; they consider that child development can only take place within the mother/child relationship (maternal function/child). The environment is the irreplaceable provider of the objects that meet the baby's basic needs. For the baby, the (metaphorical and real) support of physical contact and handling, of the reflection in the gaze of the mothering object, of the provision of objects that will make their idealization possible is indispensable. If these needs remain unmet, the development of the self will be impaired, and some of its features will be lost or altered. The self will cease to be (so) vital; it will be inharmonic and will develop certain functions while others will atrophy, or will depend on the initiative of others and will submit to them.

In this world, narcissistic but populated with objects, subjects will gradually develop a sense of self and differentiate from their fellow beings. Such progressive discrimination process requires that subjects adopt functions from early objects and have their own experiences while identifying with these objects. If everything goes well during the early stages, pathologies derived from deficit (which would appear in later years) will be avoided, but children will still have to negotiate the Oedipal phase.

Winnicott stresses his conviction that the mother-child relationship constitutes an elemental unit, and clarifies that the baby can neither be distinguished from the relationship nor be studied and interpreted as an autonomous entity. This immature baby has not yet reached the status of "autonomous centre of initiative," as Kohut describes the developed self. Neither does it have an ego with the capacity to discern its behaviours nor choose independently. As a consequence, the ability to take responsibility for its acts in general, and for aggression in particular (and the subsequent feeling of guilt), appears as a later achievement.

The notion of self takes up centre stage. The self encompasses every aspect of the person who is growing (naturally, Winnicott would say) in an environment of objects that, as I stated earlier, facilitate, support, and promote such development. They do so by performing the diverse functions described in the previous chapter, which Winnicott calls holding, handling, and object-presenting. Kohut, for his part, speaks about these objects as selfobjects. I will discuss them later. For now, I will just mention that they are absolutely necessary because they perform the functions required by human babies to relate to their own vitality and to develop their psyche. Failures at this elemental or early level result in a psychopathology grounded in absence, helplessness, object inadequacy, or overstimulation, and eventually in arrested psychological development.

The motivational forces present in these authors' conceptions are only secondarily instinctual. Both Winnicott and Kohut prioritize development needs – the search for contact and support, the potential fusion with an idealizable object, and the quest for self-affirmation. This approach leads them to claim that the most complex pathology stems not from conflict between opposing forces but from objects' failure during early stages (lack of adequate emotional response to the child's developmental needs), which becomes traumatic. Later we will see the differences between psychopathology derived from deficit and psychopathology derived from conflict. Many authors have discussed these early states and their psychopathological consequences, among them, Gedo and Goldberg (1980), Gioia (1984), Hoffmann (1999), Juri and Ferrari (2000), Killingmo (1989), Lancelle (1997), Lerner (2001), Levin de Said (1999), Modell (1984), Ortiz Frágola (1999), Painceira (1997), Paz (2005), Pelento (1992), Robbins (1983), Rodulfo (1992), Roussillon (1991), Segal (2005), Tolpin (1978), Wallerstein (1983), Zak de Goldstein (1996), Zirlinger (2001), and Zukerfeld (1999).

Winnicott and Kohut would share Fairbairn's (1941) views regarding the primal need for a meeting with the environment. As we will see later, this author considers that the libido searches for objects rather than pleasure. He posits the existence of what we could call a *primary impulse* (the search for objects as the driving force of the psyche), which diverges from Freud's notion of *secondary impulses,* according to which sexuality rests on self-conservation instincts or anaclisis. Winnicott is first and foremost a vitalist, a Buberian, while Kohut emphasizes intergenerational cooperation instead of the Oedipal struggle. Their positions are consistent with their formulations on the origin and development of the self. These two authors, as well as some of their followers, started to develop concepts hitherto not addressed by psychoanalysis, such as hope, feeling real, creativity, emptiness (as both a perception and a metapsychological concept), expressiveness, personalization (and depersonalization), and vitality. As we can see, while they start from different frames of reference and dissimilar empirical bases, Kohut and Winnicott reach similar conclusions in relation to the understanding of psychic phenomena.

Differences

I will enumerate them without thoroughly analysing them.

a   The two authors differ in the construction of their "metapsychology" and in how they modelize it. Strictly speaking, Winnicott does not resort to a particular structure. He deals neither with concepts linked to internal objects or their projections nor with secondary identifications, which Freud described so well. His main concern is authenticity –the self's creative relationship with its objects and the ability to integrate experiences. He does not try to be a metapsychologist. Nonetheless, many of the concepts he developed can be attributed metapsychological status, among them, transitional object, fantasying, creativity, use of the object, true and false self, psychopathology in terms of depressive and pre-depressive patients, and the notion of madness.[11]

Winnicott's ideas can always be deduced from clinical observation. Kohut, instead, postulates a self that can be easily represented, both in its first conception (the self as content of the Freudian psychic apparatus) and in a later version, when he proposes the idea of the self as a container of the psychic apparatus and outlines it as two poles (the pole of ideals and the pole of ambitions, which are respectively associated with "being" and "having") and, between them, a tension arc (talents and skills) that reaches from one pole to the other.

b   Another readily noticeable difference is language, that is, their style of communication. Their mode of expression does not depend only on personal traits; it is also associated with the content of their theories. Winnicott, who recreates in his language the empirical basis of his conceptualization, that is, children's play, seems light-hearted, paradoxical, and simple. His language is narrative, poetic, and singular. In 1954 he writes to Anna Freud: "I have an irritating way of saying things in my own language instead of learning how to use the terms of psychoanalytic metapsychology" (Rodman, 1987, p. 58). Kohut, whose clinical experience did not include children, uses a "scientific" language that follows a physics model (forces, poles, tension, compensation) to describe the metapsychological functioning of the self.

c   The empirical foundations are different. Winnicott opens his consultation room, and his research, to borderline personalities, psychotic patients, children, families, and mother-child pairs. Kohut, by contrast, theorizes based on his experience with patients whose pathology is close to neurosis and are affected by narcissistic disorders (which implies an already established nuclear self).

d   Their theoretical frameworks differ. Kohut's includes Freud, Hartmann, Kris, and Lowenstein, and Winnicott's, Freud, Klein, Ferenczi, Balint, Fairbairn, and Bowlby.

e   Regarding the concept of narcissism and its vicissitudes, Kohut considers that (primary object) narcissism persists throughout individuals' lives. If its development is not halted (because of pathology), it will transform, as I mentioned, into humour, wisdom, empathy, and awareness of the finitude of life. This author's description of the modes of transference that are clinically recognizable in patients with narcissistic disorders is indispensable. At first, he called them narcissistic transferences, and later, selfobject transferences, and they are the result of specific early needs. These transferences are the clinical consequence of the evolution of two developmental stages. The first involves environmental acceptance and recognition (which will appear in clinical practice as mirror transferences), and the second, the need to access ideal objects with which to blend (which will materialize in the treatment as idealizing transferences). Two selfobjects correspond to the two needs. These are the mirroring and the idealized selfobjects, which subjects experience as part of their own self.

For Winnicott, narcissism, which is always object narcissism, is based on the baby's absolute dependence on the maternal object after birth. Infants must travel the path toward independence and toward the ability to be alone. Over the course of this journey, depending on their interaction with the environment, subjects may develop a false self, which will take the shape of one of the classic psychopathological structures (borderline, schizoid, or characteropathic).[12]

f   Regarding the characteristics of the self, Kohut believes that, thanks to satisfactory experiences with its selfobjects, the self will reach its full development and will be cohesive, vital, and harmonious. Winnicott, in turn, is concerned with the difference between true (own, real, true) self, and false (adapted, foreign, impersonal) self.

g   Concerning the function of environmental objects, Kohut considers that indispensable environmental objects mirror the subject, facilitate idealization, and provide peers. Winnicott, for his part, describes an environment (in the figure of the functional environment mother) that is also absolutely necessary for the constitution and survival of the psyche in that it holds, handles, and presents objects. He describes three objects: subjective (created, envisioned, and, therefore, real for the subject), transitional (the first possession of the not-me), and objective (what is real for the social group).

h   With regard to anxiety (referred to the self), Kohut discusses the anxiety of disintegration of the self, while Winnicott addresses inconceivable anxieties (unthinkable agony) related to the fear of breakdown.

i   In relation to the continued failure of the environment, Kohut describes a defective self and argues that one pole compensates for the other pole's failure. Winnicott, in turn, refers to the *freezing* of traumatic situations when the environment impedes development. One of the pathological results is the creation of a defensive false self.

j   As to analysability, Kohut maintains that patients who suffer from narcissistic disorders and neuroses are analysable, while those who suffer from more severe pathologies are not. Winnicott, for his part, considers that severe pathologies such as schizoid and borderline disorders can be analysed, but in the case of psychoses he resorts to a technique called management.

Table 3.1 Differences between Kohut and Winnicott

Differences	*Kohut*	*Winnicott*
Language and model	"Scientific" language that outlines a metapsychology (model of the self)	"Literary" language that does not attempt to develop a metapsychology
Empirical basis of his clinical practice	Narcissistic disorders (patients with an established nuclear self)	Borderline disorders, psychotics, children, families, mother-baby couples
Theoretical framework	Freud, Hartmann, Kris, Lowenstein	Freud, Klein, Ferenczi, Balint
Narcissism	It will become empathy, humour, wisdom, acceptance of the finitude of life	Road toward independence and the ability to be alone
Features of the self	Cohesive, vital, harmonious	True vs. false (adapted)
Functions of the environment	Mirrors, makes idealization possible, provides peers	Holds, handles, and presents the object
Object	Mirroring, idealized, alter ego	Subjective, transitional, objective (real)
Consequences of the failures of needed objects	Deficit. The response: one pole compensates for the failure of the other	Trauma. Freezing of the situation. Development of a defensive false self
Analysability	In narcissism disorders and neuroses. Primary disorders of the self cannot be analysed	Analysis of borderline, schizoid and neurotic patients. In psychosis: management

I have discussed some similarities and differences between two authors who share the same perspective. Going deeper into different theoretical frameworks will certainly enable us to go farther in our search for new, more comprehensive models without misrepresenting each author's original thesis. Not only shall we avoid reductionism in our field, but it will also be easier for us to establish respectful ties with psychiatry, neuroscience, other psychologies, linguistics, anthropology, and sociology, all disciplines with which we must engage in an enriching dialogue (Table 3.1).

The patients we are seeing today in our consulting rooms, whose pathologies are increasingly complex, make it necessary for us to establish such ties. Perhaps we need to travel two parallel paths. On the one hand, we should clearly identify convergences and divergences among the various psychoanalytic perspectives; on the other, with the help of other disciplines, we should set a more comprehensive, ambitious goal that will both increase our understanding of our object of study (ultimately, our patients and our metapsychologies) and enable us to develop a symmetrical exchange with other sciences.

Notes

1 This chapter draws from the articles published in *Psicoanálisis*, 24(3): 501–520 and in *Aperturas*, three and seven, as well as from the paper presented at APdeBA's XXIII Annual Symposium in 2001, "Psiquismo temprano en el análisis de adultos: las perspectivas de Winnicott y de Kohut en el psicoanálisis actual" [Early psyche in adult analysis: Winnicott and Kohut's perspectives in present-day psychoanalysis].

2 Wallerstein (1988) and Aslan (1988) have addressed this topic. The former argues that it is clinical theory that unites us as analysts. The latter claims that the unifying foundations are psychoanalytic technique, shared theories, and analysts' personality structure.

3 Freud himself qualifies the absolute nature of these definitions, for instance, when he states as follows:

> The advance of knowledge, however, does not tolerate any rigidity even in definitions. Physics furnishes and excellent illustration of the way in which even 'basic concepts' that have been established in the form of definitions are constantly being altered in their content.
>
> (1915, p. 116)

Then, on February 15, 1924, he writes to the members of his Secret Committee that their work should be in keeping with their ideas and experiences, and that it is impossible, and not necessarily desirable, to reach full consensus among people with different temperaments. The only way they could work together, he adds, is if they all remained within the realm of shared psychoanalytic premises (Jones, 1960).

4 I argued above that perspective is always a product of the social imaginary at a certain historical juncture. Watzlawick (1976), for his part, considers that reality is a result of communication and that we distort facts so that they will not contradict our illusory perceptions of reality, instead of adapting our worldview to incontrovertible facts.

5 In fact, the e-journal *Aperturas* (www.aperturas.org), edited by Hugo Bleichmar, has been publishing research that correlates psychoanalysis and neuroscience for many years. For instance, "Las emociones vistas por el psicoanálisis y la neurociencia" [Emotions as Viewed by Psychoanalysis and Neuroscience: An Exercise in Consilience], published in 2001, narrates a research project where Panksepp, a first-rate neuroscientist who works on emotions, was asked to critically assess Freud's theory of affects in the light of his own research. Then, other neuroscientists and psychoanalysts (Antonio R. Damasio, André Green, Joseph LeDoux, Allan N. Schore, Howard Shevrin, and Clifford Yorke) were invited to consider Freud's theory and Panksepp's views from their own perspectives. This type of opening to other disciplines is highly valuable for psychoanalysts and psychiatrists.

6 Dio de Bleichmar (2002) points out that these ideas, which modify key aspects of the Freudian-Lacanian theory, show a theoretical turn in psychoanalysis. New perspectives postulate that the mind is modular, that there are multiple motivational forces organizing the psyche, and that these forces develop in parallel throughout the entire life cycle. In view of the knowledge we have acquired, only isolation and endogroup politics that tend toward consolidating the power of a few psychoanalytic schools can ignore that it is impossible to maintain simple, single-cause models in relation to the great vectors that structure the psyche. While reductive formulations are appealing because they generate a feeling of omnipotence in those who proclaim them, the concept of the complexity of interacting motivational systems is slowly making its way in psychoanalysis. These systems are attachment, hetero/self-conservation, sexuality/sensuality, and narcissism.

At the same time, we are increasingly aware of the role of aggressiveness as a defensive organization against anxieties stemming from threats to these systems, of the manifold types of unconscious processing, of the several existing memory systems, of the relationships between thematic contents processed by the mind and cross-thematic processing structures that organize these contents and are influenced by them, and so on. The linear sequencing paradigm (one stage after the other) that dominated the idea of psychic development and of the way in which association processes or psychopathological phenomena are linked has been superseded by a new conception. I am referring to parallel and distributed processing, which envisions manifold subsystems that are simultaneously active (in parallel) and emerging modules that distribute their effects through networks with specific configurations. Such specificity grants individuality to the set (McLeod et al., 1998).

7 Yet if we looked at Oedipus from the perspective of his parents' abandonment and, in that context, of Laius' vengeful murder, we would find great similarity with Hamlet.

8 Faithfulness to Freud (or to any master!) does not mean rigidly identifying with his finished products, with the letter of his writings. Instead, we should identify with his scientific journey, which involved hazarding hypotheses, rethinking ideas, and changing, integrating, discarding (Nemirovsky, 1993).

9 Papers where analysts discuss or seek to summarize an author's ideas may have different motivations and ends. It would be pathetic to present ideas simply to convince readers that the summarized theories are the only ones that finally make it possible to encompass all psychic phenomena. Leaving aside this motivation and trusting that readers will not misinterpret my goal, I am presenting here some thoughts about the reasons why I believe we must be familiar with the approaches of precursors and teachers as substantive as Winnicott and Kohut. However, we should always keep in mind that theories "are not facts, observations, or descriptions – they are organizational schemes, ways of arranging and shaping facts, observations, and descriptions" (Mitchell, 1988, p. 15).

10 As I explained in the Introduction, some situations in my clinical practice made me focus on their work. I usually treat adult patients, and also some teenagers. My basic training (at "the Lanús" and APdeBA through courses, study groups, supervisions, and my personal analyses) was Freudian and Kleinian. I relied on this framework to treat my first patients, until approximately 1982. Back then, thanks to having reached a certain maturity to face life's challenges and to my work with patients who needed something that my current notion of the setting and my own understanding of my work (my "metapsychology") could not provide, I came into contact with some authors who, in turn, referred me to others. That is how I started reading McDougall, Green, Bowlby, Erikson, and Sullivan, and to supervise with Gioia, Lancelle, and Painceira, to whom I am deeply grateful.

11 Adriana Anfusso, from Uruguay, offered me the following comment:

> Winnicott does not explicitly write about metapsychology, but when we read his work we can infer numerous metapsychological concepts, such as paradoxical thought, non-intentional aggression, regression toward dependence, the analyst's failures as opportunities, professional attitude vs. neutrality, the amorphous, the concept of use and the use of interpretation, need, self, innate potentials, the three types of object (subjective, transitional, and objective), the maternal function (holding, handling, and object-presenting), primary maternal preoccupation, primary bisexuality, existential continuity, true/false self, the three spaces (internal, transitional, and external), concern for the other, psychopathological classification, transitionality in the treatment, the notion of health, analysability, and the treatment as facilitating editions (*ediciones*).
>
> [See Translator's Note 37, Chapter 4 for an explanation
> of the choice of the word "edition" (T.N.)]

12 See Smalisnky et al. (2009) excellent book.

4   Healthiness in Winnicott and Kohut
Deficit and conflict

Donald Winnicott's concept of healthiness

As psychoanalysis evolved, the Freudian notion of healthiness (being able to love and work) gradually gave way to new criteria, which vary according to analysts' theoretical perspective on childhood development and on the organization of the psyche. Thus, just as Klein sees the integration of the object world and the working-through of mourning, as well as reparation of the damage caused to the object and subsequent gratitude, as key to define a healthy life, so does Winnicott consider that there are certain features that must be present to enjoy full well-being. These are the ability to create, to take responsibility for one's faults, and to inhabit one's body fully. He discusses these features in a variety of papers, most particularly, in "The Concept of the Healthy Individual" (1967b), where he states as follows:

> I hope that I shall not fall into the error of thinking that an individual can be assessed apart from his or her place in society. Individual maturity implies a movement towards independence, but there is no such thing as independence. It would be unhealthy for an individual to be so withdrawn as to feel independent and invulnerable. If such a person is alive, then there is dependence indeed! Dependence on mental nurse or family." The maturity Winnicott is talking about corresponds to individuals' development rather than to their chronological age, as he points out: "Premature ego development or premature self-awareness is no more healthy than is delayed awareness. The tendency towards maturation is part of that which is inherited (...) development, especially at the beginning, depends on a good-enough environmental provision (...) which facilitates the various individual inherited tendencies.
>
> (pp. 21–22)

Creativity will start at the beginning of life as long as the object is there, furnished by the environment, and adapts to the subject. The object will be there to be created by the subject. Then, the subject will have the (illusory) sense of having created the object. The (real) object will serve as an anchor for the development of creative subjectivity. The presence of the real object is a necessary condition. Yet it must be there so that subjects can create their own invention in the crossroads between the object and their experience. We should note that, particularly in relation to these descriptions, Winnicott's language is more complex than it seems. When he speaks about objective objects, he is not speaking about the real. Neither is hallucinated synonymous with subjective.

In my view, Winnicott's use of the term *hallucination* is quite unfortunate, since this term has old psychiatric roots. In some passages in *Playing and Reality* (1971) where he discusses the transitional object, he seems to ascribe to this word its traditional meaning in psychiatry; he states that the transitional object does not come from inside, and hence is not a hallucination. In *Psycho-Analytic Explorations* (1989), by contrast, he asserts that, thanks to the mother, the baby can have the illusion "that objects in external reality can be real (...) since it is only hallucinations that feel real" (Winnicott, 1989, p. 54).

The originality of this definition lies in the fact that a hallucination is the child's creation in relation to the object; it is the child's most personal, most subjective, and most characteristic aspect. Therefore, the child's perception of the object is real; for the object to be significant, the relationship with it must be a relationship with a hallucination. Only if they have hallucinated the object will subjects experience their own reality. This paradox demands that we refrain from asking whether the object was already there or was created by the subject who needed to do so. Winnicott would agree with the Spanish poet Luis Rosales, who offers an excellent definition of creation: "the invention of the non-existent necessary" (qtd. in Ridruejo, 1971, p. 407).

Hence, creativity is not a cognitive matter (a matter of "knowledge of reality"), as the sense of reality is not at play. Rather, the baby gradually creates its own objects based on already existing, material ones – on real objects.[1] If I create a world based on what I receive from the environment, life will be worth living. *Life* here is the opposite of *non-life*, which corresponds to the *living death* of schizoid, severely obsessional, and some "as if" borderline patients, rather than to the notion of death as the culmination of life processes. Creativity is thus opposed to compliance and submission, and also to the paranoid worldview that traps subjects in repetition.

Creation is always relational; we create with others, in an environment where there are others. In a meeting, correspondences, relationships are established that make new constructions visible. The creative process, therefore, subverts order. It goes against power and the revealed truth. To create also means to be unable to see the end result and to let oneself be guided by intuition. It means achieving an open-ended, unfinished structure despite the impulse to round it according to the rules of logic; one must struggle against the aesthetic appeal of closing what one perceives as open. We say we are alive if we create. Creating necessarily involves leaving our point of departure in order to reach, if possible, a different point. While we love our parents, we do not remain subordinate to them. We leave them and make our own way. We cannot say, as did the Church in the Middle Ages, "Rome has spoken, the case is closed," or resort to its equivalent for individual leaders, "*Magister dixit,*" as the last word on a topic. These expressions outline a way of thinking based on dogmatic power, which is allied to domination and is, therefore, the polar opposite of creativity.

Resorting to a theoretical perspective developed by an author (which is not expected to be homogeneous) requires using his or her ideas without fossilizing them. Winnicott warns about this danger in a letter to Klein in 1952:

> I personally think that it is very important that your work should be restated by people discovering in their own way and presenting what they discover in their own language. If you make the stipulation that in the future only your language shall be used for the statement of other people's discoveries then the language becomes a dead language (...) Your ideas will only live in so far as they are rediscovered and reformulated by original people.
>
> (Rodman, 1987, pp. 34–35)

Subjects' creativity depends (it is worth repeating) on the presence of the object. The mother must be in the right place in order to make creativity possible. As I pointed out earlier, during the last months of pregnancy and the first months of the baby's life, the mother is in a state that Winnicott calls Primary Maternal Preoccupation, a non-pathological schizoid state that drives her to adapt to the baby. This state gradually disappears "according to the baby's growing need to experience reactions to frustration" (Winnicott, 1967b, p. 22).

The idea of trauma, which I will examine further, stems from the break of continuity of existence experienced by the baby due to a failure in the environment's adaptation to its basic needs. One of those needs is to create the object. Winnicott also points out that healthiness is not the absence of illness and that, I would like to reiterate once again, health must always be assessed in relation to maturity. Maturity does not refer only to libidinal development but also to the self's ability to contain instinctive experiences and affects and to differentiate the subject from the external world.

Lasting healthiness cannot be imposed, nor can it result from negating potential feelings of unreality, of being possessed; of not being, of constantly falling; of lacking orientation; of being detached from one's body; of being nothing, nowhere. It will result, instead, from overcoming these states (which might be considered universal) with the help of an adequate environment. Health, then, encompasses experiences such as feeling alive and real, experiencing continuity in one's own existence, feeling that one is living in one's own body.

It is interesting to note something that Guntrip (1975), Winnicott's patient, repeatedly mentions about his analyst – that he had "intuitive insights." We usually define intuition as the ability to grasp the psychological situation without the intervention of theory. Intuition is a significant tool, but it needs to interact with other tools and to be conceptualized in order to become transmissible. I believe that Winnicott's insights were not just intuitive. When we come into contact with them, we appreciate that his interpretations derived from the interplay of different elements, namely, theory, the transference, the countertransference, patients' behaviour, and knowledge of their history.

I agree with Geets (1993) when he states that Winnicott's ideas only appear to be naïve. They actually point to experiences that we constantly face when treating borderline patients. Patients may experience the sense of being alive, of being real, and may experience the world as real, on the one hand, and, on the other, they may be pervaded by a feeling of being dead and by an ongoing sense of emptiness and futility, both tied to psychic death.

In present-day clinical practice, the loss of health often leads patients to tell us that they do not feel real ("I feel that everything is a movie" or "everything is happening far away from me") or that they do not feel they inhabit their own body ("I feel strange, sometimes I don't recognize myself"; or, "I don't feel it's me who is doing what I'm doing"). They often dream with endless falls, and they feel confused or that they are losing their bearings, that they "aren't anywhere." In this way, patients convey to us a sense of estrangement that is often accompanied by reduced sensitivity and a difficulty to express their feelings (alexithymia). The consequences of these feelings on self-esteem are remarkable. When patients start regaining their health during a treatment, the restoration of these functions and its emotional repercussions (a feeling of plenitude, of "wanting to live life") are obvious.

Heinz Kohut's concept of health

In Chapter 2, I pointed out Kohut's contention that if human infants' development is not halted by traumatic events (basically, if the environment supports them by meeting their development needs), their self will be cohesive, vital, and harmonious. Cohesion will result from the absence of structural dissociation (the opposite result is the fragmentation of the self), while vitality will be the driving force that will facilitate the pursuit of goals and ideals. Children will be able to endure or overcome obstacles or, if these are unconquerable, to wait and resume their search at the right time without losing their creative impulses, without which they would fall into indifference or depression. Harmony between the poles configuring the self will give rise to a balanced personality, which is an expression of maturity.

From Kohut's perspective, health is the product of an environment constituted by selfobjects that can respond to the child's needs with their presence, attentive listening, silent serenity, and quiet mirroring, and that can fail adequately. In other words, these objects can gradually cease to perform their functions when subjects are ready to respond to such failures with a transmuting internalization (by introjecting object functions). From this perspective, individuals' sense of self derives from an everyday experience, that is, the sense of an integrated existence. Subjects perceive themselves as real and as agents of their actions. They are able to feel, have intentions, develop plans, express themselves through language, and share personal experiences. Health also involves the experience of intimacy.

Kohut develops these concepts, which are so valuable for our clinical practice today, in his second book (*The Restoration of the Self*, in Chapter III, the section titled "The Psychoanalyst's Child"). There, he describes adult patients who experience the feeling of not being real and need to attach themselves to powerful figures in order to feel alive. While neither cold nor rejecting, these patients' parents acted intrusively, early on, by offering "interpretations" about what their children thought, wished, and felt. As a result, these patients experienced difficulties in consolidating their self and defensively adopted a secret, isolated life to prevent their parents' intrusion.

We should recall here that unlike Freud, Kohut does not view human psychic development as finite; it does not end with the consolidation of an "apparatus" that processes drives. As I mentioned in Chapter 2, he is fighting against a prejudice according to which narcissism is more primitive, and object relations, more evolved. From this perspective, the cure would depend on the transformation of narcissism into object libido to achieve maturity. We should also stress that, as an alternative to Freudian thought, Kohut postulates two independent development paths that are equally valuable, namely, the narcissism route and the instinct-object route. Narcissism can gradually transform into a healthy component of the self.

Kohut clarifies, however, that he does not define narcissism based on the type of object with which subjects relate or on the charge with which these objects are invested, but on the type of bond. This narcissistic way of relating to objects, which at first sees the object as part of the self (selfobject), will be enriched and will transform, and it is a key aspect of every commitment to a bond. It will change until it will eventually generate empathy (the ability to put oneself in the other's place, and thus to understand), wisdom, humour, and the acceptance of the finitude of life.

Deficit and conflict

When we speak of deficit (especially if we look at it from the perspective of Freud's second topography), we probably have in mind the failed structuring and consolidation of the three agencies (ego, superego, and ego ideal) as mature formations. A weak ego resorts to dissociation rather than to repression, has a low tolerance to frustration, and shows perception and self-perception disorders as well as a lack of control over impulses and a tendency to develop fantasy life rather than real life. The superego oscillates between severe punishment and inaction, and therefore its interventions are unpredictable. Last, the ego ideal (the ideals put forward by the superego) is also poorly developed, and the values it supports are fragile, thence a common tendency toward hasty idealization and prompt disappointment. For this reason, self-esteem disorders are common.

These failures are caused by pre-Oedipal disorders (in the bond with early objects), a notion that refers to a genetic-developmental model similar to the one Freud (1926) formulates in "Inhibitions, Symptom and Anxiety." This model is based on the concept of developmental line set forth by Ferenczi, who describes the dangers of psychic helplessness corresponding to each period of psychic immaturity. These dangers are the trauma of birth and the loss of the needed object at the beginning of life; the danger of castration during the phallic phase; and later, when development has progressed further, the anxiety concerning the superego during the latency period, with a progressive increase in tension and an inability to dominate it, both characteristic of the state of helplessness.[2]

In *The Language of Psychoanalysis*, Laplanche and Pontalis state that helplessness (*Hilflosigkeit*)

> has a specific meaning in Freudian Theory, where it is used to denote the state of the human suckling which, being entirely dependent on other people for the satisfaction of its needs (hunger, thirst), proves incapable of carrying out the specific action necessary to put an end to internal tension. For the adult, the state of helplessness is the prototype of the traumatic situation which is responsible for the generation of anxiety.
> (Laplanche and Pontalis, 1973, p. 189)

This is the prototype of the traumatic situation. From a Freudian perspective, then, deficit implies structural failure. From the perspective of authors who are mainly concerned with the development of the self, the notion of deficit refers to a self with a deficient structure. This self resembles a kaleidoscope configured by manifold splits, and the clinical consequences are the following:

identity diffusion;
lack of object constancy;
self-esteem disturbances;
disturbances in the regulation of anxiety; and
especially in schizoid subjects, a decrease in vitality and in the acknowledgment of desire.

These patients are clinically heterogeneous. I cannot provide a specific description, but many of them have struck me as automatons, as living dead, especially during the periods when they are not involved in any "action." The typical problem they display in their object relations is bipersonal rather than triangular. Faced with a mourning situation, moreover, they fragment or collapse. They usually present with monotonous speech, and provoke irritation or boredom when they are not suffering a temporary passionate outburst. What predominates is fragmentation anxiety – a fear of ceasing to be, of disappearing without warning.

Deficit appears clinically as a feeling of emptiness and unreality and as an ever-present fear of breakdown, of imminent fragmentation of variable intensity. These feelings bring into play a series of mechanisms aimed at survival. Sexuality becomes secondary and is sometimes used defensively. That is why Joyce McDougall states that in these patients,

> Narcissus plays a more important role than Oedipus (...) psychic survival occupies a more fundamental place (...) than the Oedipal crisis, to the extent that for some suffering occasioned by the question of sexual rights and desires takes on the appearance of a luxury.
>
> (1978, p. 302)

The survival alluded to by McDougall constitutes an attempt to satisfy the needs of the self.

Table 4.1, based on Killingmo (1989) and modified from Aguilar (2000), is intended to summarize the foregoing explanation.

Table 4.1 Conflict and Deficit

Characteristics	Conflict	Deficit
Origin	Intrasystemic	Intersubjective (Structural deficit: lack of object constancy, identity diffusion, enfeebled ego, devitalization of desire, low self-esteem)
Motivation	Structural conflicts (among agencies, identifications, internal objects)	Environmental failure to meet needs due to neglect, abuse, absence. Traumas, pathological identifications
Basic mechanism	Repression	Dissociation
Individuation	Self/object differentiation is present	Poor self/object differentiation
Type of anxiety	Castration anxiety	Breakdown anxiety (due to fragmentation of the self)
Treatment: type of prevailing intervention	Interpretation of transference repetition *per via di levare* (seeks to reveal hidden contents)[3]	Affirmative interventions: give meaning, understand *per via di creare*.[4] They need to *edit*[5] the experience

What follows is an outline of the self's needs (and it should be emphasized once again that they must be met in order to make psychic development possible):

- being supported, mirrored, understood;
- being able to idealize an object and fuse with it with confidence and constancy in order to share its capacities (ability to tolerate and modulate emotions);
- feeling equal or similar to other humans. The deficit resulting from the subject's bonds with these fellow beings will generate one of the following transferences: mirror, idealizing, or twinship (Kohut's nomenclature);
- Winnicott postulates that one of the baby's basic needs is for the mother to guess what it needs, whereas with the onset of the transition state, the prevalent need is to have its intimacy respected;
- perhaps there are many other needs left to describe. Let us say once again that meeting them is as essential as environmental factors are for the development of living beings, and that they are usually satisfied or mitigated in psychoanalytic treatment by way of the setting and our analytic attitude. Multiple elements are critical to this process, from our presence to the phonological aspects of speech (the tone, pitch, and rhythm of our utterances).

The developmental stages of children's needs cannot be skipped or replaced. Moreover, they represent intersubjective milestones in each phase of the life cycle. Babies and children's development will depend on the quality of the support they receive, of the mirroring they experience – of the complementarity of the earliest objects. Needs cannot be frustrated, for the notion of frustration is reserved for conflicting drives. If needs are not met, they will remain frozen until the environment makes their development possible.

As we can see, the problems leading to pathological development precede the Oedipal (libidinal or aggressive) conflict. Different authors speak of different needs. Winnicott (1965a) postulates the need to maintain the continuity of being, and designates as *trauma* any interruption of the child's "going on being." Mahler and her colleagues speak of symbiotic fusion (Mahler et al., 1975), while Kohut (1971) points out that met needs enable babies to affirm their basic sense of self.[6] The self may be damaged (become helpless) because of the presence of an intrusive object or the absence of the needed objects at a time when the self is unable to represent causes and effects and has not yet become an "independent centre of initiative." In this case, the consequences will be vague feelings of confusion, shame, and guilt that fragment the self. Defences, therefore, will be aimed at avoiding such fragmentation. In clinical practice, the entire process translates as depersonalization.

These deficient structures tend to be accompanied by, and combine with, the effects of psychic conflict. Nevertheless, deficient structures (which may be identified as the treatment progresses) always lead us to formulate hypotheses regarding their cause. I have already mentioned that Fairbairn (1941) suggests that the libido seeks objects rather than pleasure, that erogenous zones are mediating channels, and that libidinal phases are "ego techniques" that serve to regulate object relations. In this way, the foundations are laid for a conception of a "primary impulse" (the search for objects as the main driving force of the psyche), a conception that differs from that of "secondary impulses" advocated by Freud. As I mentioned earlier, according to the latter conception, sexuality rests on the instincts (anaclisis).

If we adopt Fairbairn's depiction of the libido (as seeking objects rather than pleasure) and connect it with the notion of the self as the individual's psychological centre, we can see that the psychoanalysis of neuroses leaves out not just the bodily, organic aspects of development ("self-conservation"), but also an entire world of early bonds that does not have a place in classic metapsychology. Patients who seek our help nowadays have doubts about themselves, about their identity. Many of them display a state of empty depression and experience feelings of futility, senselessness, hopelessness, apathy, and emotional numbness. They set erratic or compulsive goals for themselves, and need contact with others, a need that usually drives them to be promiscuous or indiscriminate in their sex life.

We could claim that the driving force behind some complex behaviours that are manifestly sexual, such as "perverse" episodes of acting out, borderline patients' sexual acting out, or compulsive sexuality, is the need (of a precarious self) to attain cohesiveness, integration, or contact – an essentially narcissistic problem[7] that is viewed as an Oedipal conflict. These patients with deficit pathologies try to find objects that will offer them the modes of satisfaction they are primarily seeking (support, mirroring, attachment, constancy, calm, intimacy, and so on). Analysts' main goal will not be to reveal or uncover, but to help the self experience its own existence. These patients are not trying to find something in order to possess it, but to feel they exist.

They also tend toward depersonalization, and experience the following:

1   Situations of estrangement regarding one's own body: location disorders (living outside one's body, or feeling split), distortion in body-image boundaries, in body awareness, and in the estimation of the size of body parts.
2   Feelings of unreality, emptiness, futility, senselessness: feeling that one is "inside a dream," that one is an automaton, a robot, numb. These feelings are accompanied by depressive affects without self-reproach.
3   Disturbance of the sense of evidence, that is, déjà-vu and jamais-vu phenomena. Doubts about what one knows or sees; lack of conviction in the face of the evidence.
4   Affects accompanying the experience: perplexity, uncertainty, "distress."

Patients resort to the following techniques to control depersonalization: self-stimulation (masturbation, drinking strong drinks or spicy food, drugs, violent workout, risky sports, self-provoked fear or vertigo); unusual use of the senses (smelling parts of one's own body to recognize oneself); listening to music to recover; touching oneself as a ritual; hurting or beating oneself, or driving one's nails into the palms of one's hands; concealment, especially behind paranoid defences.

Hoffmann (1984) has thoroughly studied this matter. This author points out that in theories of the self, acute depersonalization is as significant as signal anxiety is for classic psychoanalytic theory (Freud, 1926). The phenomena described above may be found especially in narcissistic (Kohut's Narcissistic Personality Disorder), schizoid (Fairbairn, Winnicott), "pre-genital phobic" (Bouvet, 1968), depressive, and panicky patients, and in those who are undergoing pathological or acute mourning. Depersonalization implies a threat to integrity, to temporal continuity, and to the self's sense of cohesion. It can become part of subjects' personality and generate a chronic form of fragmentation or disintegration that is perceived as an ongoing sense of foreignness.

Hugo de Saint Victor, a twelfth-century Saxon monk, expresses this state poetically: "He who finds his motherland sweet is a noble apprentice; he who finds that every land is a native land is already strong; but perfect is the one for whom the entire world is foreign" (qtd in Kozer, 2005, p. 31). The emotional states inherent in depersonalization are hard to convey, particularly because they demand a complex use of metaphor that is not always available to the patient. Analysts grasp these states based on their countertransference, which plays a key role in the understanding of complex patients.

Some aspects of the setting and of interpretation in these pathologies

For those (deficit) patients who need it as a "specific action," the setting will be the means by which analysts provide the specialized environment that will enable patients, by their making use of it, to develop in the transference aspects of the self that had frozen in childhood. We should recall here the epigraph of Chapter 2, where Winnicott (1955) alerts us to the inescapable need to study adaptation if we want our discipline to develop further. Today, many of our patients need a carefully arranged setting that will provide them with a metaphor, a replica, or substitute for maternal care, so that they can experience a new edition; they have never experienced, and hence have not appropriated, a setting for their everyday life.[8] They need this edition in order to continue with their development. I call *edition* the mechanism whereby the psyche may develop, thanks to a meeting between two subjects – one who is willing to trust, and the other who is available to respond with a specific action. This meeting may give rise to the (neo)formation of hitherto non-existent psyche. I explain this concept in depth in Chapter 7.[9]

For this type of transference to unfold, the right setting must be established, a setting that will be specific to each patient. Concerning the setting/transference relationship, Puget (1991) states: "While the 'classic' theory of the transference assumes that everything can be transferred, not everything can," and adds: "the transference cannot unfold because the setting is inadequate" (Puget, 1991, p. 400). In this way, Puget prioritizes the setting-patient equation, whose result will be a setting that, by facilitating the unfolding of the transference, renders the psychoanalytic process viable.[10]

Regarding interpretation, it is worth highlighting the specific traits displayed by patients with a structural deficit. While our work with conflict involves helping them face their impulses and reveal hidden meanings (*via di levare*), when patients present with a deficit we should allow them to experience a sense of self. Rather than finding something they have lost, patients should feel that something exists, as Killingmo (1989) argues. This author advocates "affirmative interventions" (which he opposes to "interpretive interventions," suitable to tackle conflict). These are aimed to discern self and object representations as well as diffuse or distorted self perceptions so that patients can internalize object relations, something they had not been able to do in the past.

We try to promote patients' ability to perceive what belongs to them, thus confirming the validity of their experience. This type of affirmative intervention may bear varying degrees of complexity and generally includes containment and support. In this way, we favour giving meaning to patients' experiences with both words and silences. We try to create rather than reveal meaning. Before Killingmo, Meltzer (1975) comes close to this approach when, in his analysis of adhesive identification, he posits the absence of an internal object and the need to create it. This author claims that we cannot fill a hole by digging, in reference to the ineffectiveness in these cases of interpretations *per via di levare*.

I pointed out earlier that Lerner and I have called *need transference* the transference born from structural deficit (Lerner and Nemirovsky, 1990). When making affirmative interventions, we must empathize with patients' affects as much as we can while working with an open field of signification so that we do not assert that patients are sad when they are actually in a depressive mood. Instead, we should suggest a "menu" of options in order to find the affective resonance most syntonic with them. Patients should choose the word that most resembles their emotional state (we could suggest different synonyms, such as sad, low, or lethargic). We should do the same, furthermore, if we encountered poorly discriminated feelings of anger (wrath, rage, fury, anger).

Winnicott repeatedly stresses the baby's right to have the mother guess how it feels through primary maternal preoccupation. Perhaps it is analysts' emotional availability, a metaphor of that early (and likely failed) relationship with the mother, that will come to their aid. It would be utopian to attribute to those analysts who have an emotional disposition to understand patients' states the maternal qualities involved in the state of maternal preoccupation. Nonetheless, the analyst's position will be isomorphic with that of the mother who is preoccupied with her child during its early years. Such isomorphism is associated with the ethical position that analysts must adopt in order to work with these pathologies.

Notes

1 William Blake (1906, p. 13) wrote: "A fool sees not the same tree that a wise man sees," where "to see" refers not to what is perceived but to what is created. The word *Erlebnis* (experience) used by Dilthey and Husserl corresponds to our notion.

2 According to Freud (1926), as the human being is "sent into the world in a less than finished state," the external world has a greater influence on it. Consequently, "the dangers of the external world have a greater importance for it, so that the value of the object which can alone protect it against them [...]. The biological factor, then, establishes the earliest situations of danger and creates the need to be loved which will accompany the child through the rest of his life" (Freud, 1926, pp. 168–169).

3 The author refers to Freud's (1905) comparison between psychoanalysis and suggestion. Rather than *"per via da porre"* (by adding), as painting does, psychoanalysis, like sculpture, works *"per via di levare"*; it takes away what covers the surface ("On Psychotherapy," *S. E.*, **7**: 255–268). (T.N.)

4 Concerning the *via di creare*, see the final paragraphs of Chapter 9.

5 I provide a brief definition of *edition* (*edición*) in the next section. See Chapter 7 for a more detailed explanation of this concept [See T.N. 37 for an explanation of the choice of the term in English (T.N.)].

6 Winnicott often stresses that psychotic anxiety is tied to the failure to satisfy basic needs. For instance, in a letter to Lili Peller in 1966, he writes that psychotic anxieties "have nothing to do with instincts. They have to do with such things as disintegration, depersonalisation (...) annihilation, falling for ever, lack of contact with not-me objects, etc." (Rodman, 1987, p. 56). We should relate this statement to the Freudian concept of helplessness.

7 I use narcissism in Kohut's sense of the term. As I pointed out earlier, I take as a parameter *the quality of the object relation*. The narcissistic bond with the selfobject renders the latter indispensable for the constitution, harmony, and continuity of the self. This object is part of the self, and its absence or estrangement does not trigger mourning but a breakdown.

8 It should be noted that the setting (if it includes one's professional attitude) does not allow us to replace what was literally not there. It recreates a bond (if everything goes well); it creates a unique, original atmosphere.

9 The author chose to translate the words *"edición"* and *"reedición"* as *edition* and *re-edition*, despite the difference in usage between Spanish and English, in order to highlight the novelty of the concept. (T.N.)

10 At present, due to the nature of our times, the ability to develop a stable setting is exceptional. (Even though many psychoanalytic institutes still teach that this is the setting that should be established, as though by overlooking the current features of our work, we could illusorily recreate the frame used decades ago.) The demand for treatment is gradually increasing in all social sectors and, more than ever, we need to have a clear analytic attitude that will allow us to create a space of reflection in the timeline and spatial conditions that are available to us. Today we see patients every other week, often once a week, and exceptionally two or more times a week. We also exchange emails with them and analyse them over the phone. In addition, we are often asked to change the time and day of the sessions, mostly at the last minute, and patients absent themselves for long periods of time.

5   Trauma after Freud

In a conception that we could call traditional, trauma is an event in the subject's life defined by its intensity, by the subject's incapacity to respond adequately to it, and by the upheaval and long-lasting effects that it brings about in the psychical organization. In economic terms, the trauma is characterized by an influx of excitations that is excessive by the standard of the subject's tolerance and capacity to master such excitations and work them out psychically. (Laplanche and Pontalis, 1973, p. 465).

Among Argentine authors, Benyakar (2003, p. 42) defines disruptive events as "any event or situation that has the potential to invade the psyche and provoke reactions that alter its capacity to integrate and work through."

Freud initially considers trauma an economic issue tied to seduction (the amount of excitation reaching the psyche that exceeds its capacity to tolerate stimuli). Yet this conception gradually changes as he tries to explain what seems evident in his practice. Thus, in the first, pre-psychoanalytic period (1890–1897) he attributes the cause of neurosis to early traumas that are specific to subjects' history, can be located in time, and are not necessarily of a sexual nature, such as the loss of a loved one or being abandoned by someone. These traumas were not experienced under a situation of psychological weakness (for instance, a hypnoid state, as Breuer called it), and cannot be "discharged" through abreaction. For this reason, they keep generating pathogenic effects.

As he delves into the study of hysteria, Freud inevitably narrows the genesis of trauma to a sexual, prepubescent origin. An event that takes place during childhood (for instance, seduction by an adult) provokes no reaction, but with the blossoming of sexuality during puberty, it appears through retroactive reactivation (*après-coup*), with its emotional correlate. According to this second theory, endogenous factors (what must be contributed by the subject for the trauma to be effective) acquire greater weight. At this stage, the notion of disposition due to libido fixation (heredity shaped by childhood events) is clearly established, as well as the onset of hysteria due to an accidental, traumatic factor. This development implies the appearance of frustration in the aetiology of neuroses. In Freud's fully developed metapsychology, fantasy plays a critical role. We no longer need an actual, effective event to generate a trauma; it is the nature of fantasy life itself that predisposes subjects for the acquisition of traumata.

In *Beyond the Pleasure Principle* (1920) Freud recreates ideas originally discussed in the *Project for a Scientific Psychology* (1950 [1895]). He conceives of the organism as shielded from external stimuli by a protecting layer that only lets tolerable amounts of excitation through. These original ideas about trauma are considerably expanded by the formulations advanced in "Inhibitions, Symptoms and Anxiety" (1926) in relation to signal anxiety. As Laplanche and Pontalis point out, "This account in effect postulates a kind of diametrical opposition between the external danger and the internal one: the ego is attacked from within – that is to say, by instinctual excitations – *just as* it is from without" (Laplanche and Pontalis, 1973, p. 469; authors' emphasis).

Here, he describes the dangers that children must avoid over the course of their development. As I mentioned earlier, he follows a model of development based on risk stages. Freud situates these (epigenetic) dangers, which could result in traumatic situations, at specific developmental stages. Ferenczi (1933) will be the one to develop these formulations. He will postulate that trauma is the consequence of the object's failure to provide an adequate response to a situation of helplessness. (These ideas will be the basis of what we might call the Psychology of Deficit, upon which Winnicott and Kohut will build, following the Hungarian School pioneers.)

While Freud laid the foundations for these ideas in 1926, when he posited the epigenetic development of anxiety, Ferenczi was, perhaps, the one who formulated the most original conception of trauma. As it is usually the case, while several authors may share the same perspective, one of them appears as the innovator because he or she synthesizes ideas that are circulating in his or her scientific milieu (anonymous ideas). Concerning this particular subject, there are multiple "debts," such as the ones Winnicott owes Ferenczi and the ones later authors, among them, Kohut, Mitchell, Orange, and Stolorow, owe the first two.

Already in 1933, Ferenczi had highlighted the relevance, undisputed today, of violence and sexual abuse in the aetiology of mental pathologies. His viewpoint was dismissed, however, because Kleinian analysts favoured the notion of fantasy. At that stage in the history of psychoanalysis, prevailing theories considered that psychic life was confined to the realm of fantasy and overlooked the circumstances of subjects' lives. As Laplanche (1987) points out, Freud's abandonment of the seduction theory led to the prevalence of an endogenist perspective that focused on the drives and did not take into account the role of the environment in their development.

The above-mentioned perspectives may be clearly distinguished from those propounded by Klein and the Kleinian school, which followed Abraham. For these authors, the essential threat is posed by internal sources rather than by the absence of the object or primary object failures – it is the threat of the death drive, originating in one's own psyche, that will give rise to traumatic situations. Other members of the British school, such as Bowlby (1951), link trauma to the inability to develop an adequate attachment relationship. This author found that many children deprived of their parents during World War II suffered greatly because of this absence.

It is worth considering here Valeros's (2005) ideas regarding Bowlby's notion of trauma:

> Yet this somewhat simple, almost physicalistic conception of attachment trauma was gradually combined with another, more functional aspect of the attachment bond, that is, the psychological quality of this bond. Bowlby gradually recognized that the significance of attachments is also tied to the presence and physical proximity of the attachment figure – what he called the mother's "sensitivity" to her bond with the child. By "sensitivity," Bowlby understood the mother's capacity to understand, to empathize with her child's emotional states and to respond accordingly.
>
> (Valeros, 2005, pp. 205–206)

For Bowlby, this special bond includes the attachment figure's physical availability and the quality of his or her empathic response. Any significant disturbance of these two factors predisposes the child for a traumatic situation.

So far, I have summarized only one vertex of Bowlby's ideas, that is, the child's interpersonal relationship with the mother. Now I must focus on the other vertex of the attachment bond – the child's internalization of the features of this bond. Bowlby (1969) calls such internalization the "working model" of the attachment bond. His intrapsychic model of the relationship with the mother is similar to the one advanced by object relations theory. There is a difference, however, that he highlights. The two models are based on different hypotheses about the origin and content of the system of relations in the internal world. According to Bowlby, working models of the attachment bond are a faithful representation of the actual qualities of the bond between mother and child. At the same time, his view is diametrically opposed to psychoanalytic theories according to which fantasies about object relations are the result of endogenous processes disconnected from subjects' relationship with real attachment figures.

Going back to Bowlby's concept of trauma, we should stress that he postulates an interdependent dynamic interaction between external trauma, the quality of attachment in internal models, and the availability of attachment figures that may help work through that trauma. On the other side of the ocean is Kohut, the creator of the psychology of the self. Let us set aside the concepts that preceded his original developments on the nature of narcissistic bonds, and focus on the relationship between the developing baby and its selfobjects. As we saw earlier, these objects' inadequate (absent or excessive) response to the evolving self's mirroring and idealizing needs has a traumatic effect. If such failure persists, moreover, it will result in defective psychic structures. We are, therefore, a long way from optimal frustration, which involves a disappointment that matches the baby's stage of development and leads to the transmuting internalization of experiences undergone with selfobjects.

As Lancelle (1984) points out,

> Kohut develops the concept of trauma before his theory of narcissism and his psychology of the self, but his conclusions about it are later applied to his conception of the self. As early as 1963, along with Seitz, Kohut describes trauma as the key factor in the development of psychopathology, a thesis he ratifies in his studies on narcissism and on the psychology and psychopathology of the self. Childhood trauma is an emotional situation that the child's psyche cannot integrate into the differentiated preconscious because the demand is too intense, the structures are too immature, or the psyche is transitorily hypersensitive.
>
> (Lancelle, 1984, p. 453)

Kohut (1971) also talks about traumatic frustrations. Frustrations are traumatic when they surpass the psyche's tolerance or when gratifications are intense and unpredictable. This author argues that therapists can handle childhood frustrations if the latter is activated within the therapeutic situation in acceptable degrees. Their gradual working-through, moreover, facilitates the development of the psychic structure.

Trauma, self, neutrality

In the framework of the concept of self, the notion of trauma acquires specific features. The formation of the self is gradual, and it is polarized around two types of structuring experiences that I described earlier – mirroring and idealizing experiences. The baby's interaction with objects that provide suitable responses to its needs (selfobjects) will give rise to the poles of ambitions and ideals as well as to the goals that configure the personality. Through inevitable, but non-traumatic, disappointment with these objects, the self-object relationship is replaced by the child's psychic structure, as long as, precisely, these disappointments are not traumatic.

In self psychology, optimal frustration corresponds to these non-traumatic disappointments, that is, series or sequences of events occurring in the child's experience with its selfobjects, which, in relative terms, fail to respond to its needs. The self can assimilate such failures as long as they do not affect its cohesion. Rather than repressing or disassociating the experience of frustration, the self undergoes an internalization process whereby the relationship with the selfobject becomes psychic structure that substitutes for the object's functions. For example, the (hetero)esteem of an object that accepts and mirrors gradually leads to the development of self-esteem.

Chronic traumatic states are associated with disorders of the self (narcissistic personality disorders and narcissistic behaviour disorders). When narcissistic structures are weak, the self is markedly exposed to transitory fragmentation in the face of disappointment or of a faulty empathic environment. Trauma may affect the development of the grandiose self and the idealized parental imago, the two primitive structures of the nuclear self. Under the impact of a severe trauma, neither of these structures integrates into the personality, and their demands are perpetuated. Such narcissistic configurations are relatively stable and may be relived in the therapeutic relationship, thanks to transference experiences corresponding to each configuration. Kohut gives the name of *narcissistic transferences* (or, in his last publications, *transferences with selfobjects*) to the clinical reactivations of these configurations. *Mirror transference* corresponds to the clinical phenomenon that activates the grandiose self, and *idealizing transference*, to the one that activates the idealized parental imago.

Reflecting on what non-neurotic patients experience as traumatic inevitably leads us to the notion of analytic neutrality, which does not pose an obstacle to the treatment of patients whose pathology derives from the Oedipus complex. In the name of a poorly understood analytic neutrality, analysts often stay silent and offer no answer or explanation to patients' requirements or questions. Coldness and emotional distance are never appropriate or neutral. What is more, especially with patients who have experienced early suffering, they favour the repetition of traumatic experiences with childhood selfobjects.

Laplanche and Pontalis are categorical: "The analyst must be *neutral* in respect of religious, ethical and social values – that is to say, he must not direct the treatment according to some ideal" (Laplanche and Pontalis, 1973, p. 271; authors' emphasis). For a start, neutrality, on the contrary, means providing the average response (Hartmann, 1970) expectable from a fellow being. We must, therefore, reject the idea of "non-participation." Their analytic attitude is neutral when, by putting themselves in their patient's shoes, analysts understand that they should not provoke reactions in their patients.

I agree with Renik's (2002, p. 497) considerations on this issue:

> The concept of analytic neutrality has become a burden in that it encourages us to perpetuate certain limiting illusions about the analyst's role in the psychoanalytic process. I propose to criticize the concept of analytic neutrality in three ways:
> 1 It does not take account of the way learning actually takes place in analysis, and therefore does not describe the ideal relation between an analyst's judgements and a patient's conflicts.
> 2 It suggests a misguided view of the role of the analyst's emotions in analytic technique.

3   It is part of an erroneous conception of the domain of analytic technique, and therefore contributes to a misunderstanding of what deters analysts from exploitation of patients.

Renik argues that regardless of analysts' self-analysis, there will be unconscious factors that will influence our observations and interventions. Analysts, he claims, cannot avoid being subjective, and that is why we must establish technical principles that will mitigate the effects of this subjective condition. In addition, silence may be the consequence of a misunderstanding of the notion of neutrality. Excessive distance, in fact, is the opposite of neutrality, and may generate reactions in our patients that repeat the cycle of childhood traumatic experiences.

This sequence could serve as an example: child's curiosity → lack of an adequate response on the part of early objects, which is experienced as disapproval → child's reaction → early objects' reproachful reaction → traumatic inhibition of curiosity. A lack of understanding of this technical concept will probably affect analysts' ability to understand their patients by way of an open intersubjective exchange. We may deceive ourselves if we do not approach clinical psychoanalysis as a dialectical process between two participants, neither of whom is actually neutral.

Trauma and parental personality

Kohut (1977) states that although disagreements between the parents provoke great fear, the suffering due to subtle absences of parents or caregivers is worse when such absences result from an empty personality or non-manifest psychosis. Caregivers' emptiness leads to the worst possible suffering, while their hidden psychosis causes them to ignore the reality of the child's existence and treat the child as a thing or as an extension of themselves. It creates an "anaerobic" environment. These children are unable to distinguish between good and bad care because they assume that the environment where they are growing up is normal. They feel deeply guilty for wishing for what their caregivers cannot give them. Some classically described traumas, such as witnessing the primal scene, must be considered pathogenic not because of undue witnessing but because they are clues to parental neglect or indifference.

Ferenczi often refers to traumatic situations tied to parental personality issues. In 1929 he writes that we should realize how sensitive children are, even if the parents believe otherwise and act in their offspring's presence as if their own behaviour had no effect on the children. At the same time, Winnicott's thoughts on this matter are connected with his ideas concerning the "line of development" of children's dependence on their early environmental objects. If environmental failures (during the journey that goes from absolute dependence to relative independence in relation to the maternal object) are significant and ongoing (due to absence, intrusion, or abuse), they will result in arrested development, thus causing a break in the child's existential continuity. A possible consequence is forced mental adaptation, the source of the false self.

If these potentially traumatic failures occur during the earliest subjectivation stage, they will not be perceived as an experience but will remain "catalogued" or "frozen," waiting for a meeting that will facilitate their appearance and edition. Such halts in development can only be vividly experienced in specific bond situations. In these situations, an environment is created (analysis may be a favourable environmental situation, depending on the analyst's attitude!) in which patients who were traumatized in their early childhood may feel certain that their current surroundings are the product of their own projection (based on the exercise of the omnipotence that was aborted during the phase of absolute dependence).

How are these early traumas expressed in the patient's psychic structure and in the transference? From this perspective, phenomena such as depersonalization and estrangement, so frequent in our consulting rooms today and ever-present components of countless clinical pictures (panic attacks, borderline personalities, onset of schizophrenia, severe neurosis), would be current manifestations of early traumatic situations caused by the lack of a necessary environmental response. (These pictures usually include feelings that were also acquired early in life, such as endlessly falling, losing contact with one's own body, disorientation, or bodily fragmentation.) As I pointed out earlier, Winnicott summarized such response with the notions of holding, handling, and object-presenting, which should be present during the upbringing of human infants.

Regarding the transference, Winnicott states that what the patient needs

is to remember the original madness, but in fact the madness belongs to a very early stage before the organization in the ego of those intellectual processes which can abstract experiences that have been catalogued and can present them for use in terms of conscious memory. In other words madness that has to be remembered can only be remembered in the reliving of it (...) the aim of the patient [is] (...) to be mad in the analytic setting, the nearest the patient can ever do to remembering.

(Winnicott, 1989, p. 125)

Later he adds that these patients have already had the breakdown they so fear, and what we identify as their current illness is a defence system that has been organized in relation to that breakdown. The fear of breakdown is rooted in the need to recall the original traumatic situation. When this breakdown is experienced for the first time, it can be edited to be remembered later. "Behind such a breakdown there is always (...) a failure of defences belonging to the individual's infancy or very early childhood" (Winnicott, 1960b, p. 139). I will come back to these concepts later.

We should recall here that when Winnicott (1962) wonders what is a baby, he is not referring to the dimension of the drives. He does not view the baby as someone who is hungry and "whose instinctual drives may be met or frustrated." Rather, he highlights that the baby is "an immature being who is all the time on the brink of unthinkable anxiety" (p. 57). This particular form of anxiety, which is unthinkable, refers in the adult to feelings of fragmentation, fall, loss of one's relationship to one's body, disorientation, and isolation. The maternal function keeps it at bay. As the ego matures, it gradually takes control, allowing these feelings to move to the background.

The epigraph of this book quotes Rickman's comment to Winnicott: "Insanity is not being able to find anyone to stand you." For tolerance to happen, Winnicott continues, "there are two factors: the degree of illness in the patient and the ability of the environment to tolerate the symptoms" (Winnicott, 1961, p. 109). And in a later essay he states: "Relaxation for an infant means not feeling a need to integrate, the mother's ego-supporting function being taken for granted" (Winnicott, 1962, p. 61). Integration is closely tied to the environmental function of *holding*. During a treatment, holding is in direct relationship to the analyst's behaviour, which is represented by the frame, the setting, and must be adapted to patients' needs.

Holding, however, will only be possible if patients trust their analysts' behaviour and set aside their defences, and if analysts accept patients' fusional transference, which places the analyst in the position of a subjective object. Only then will the early situation that was traumatically interrupted be recreated. It is worth mentioning that sooner or later, and inevitably, analysts will fail. If everything goes well, contrary to what happens in the case of pathogenic failure, the analytic frame and attitude will contain the analyst's failure and give the patient the opportunity to (re)live the original trauma in a safe, non-retaliating, non-reactive environment. It is only in this type of environment that the right conditions will develop for the edition of hitherto frozen (new) psychic structures (C. Nemirovsky, 1999, 2003).

Roussillon (1991) uses the term *pre-psychic traumas* for those traumas that have not been edited because no psychic representation of the traumatic experience exists at this time. The subject was not there to create a representation because the trauma preceded subjectivation. What remains is absence, lack, the negative. "Since it is not an experience proper, the traumatic is not constituted as memory and, therefore, cannot be remembered or forgotten" (Jordán, 2001, p. 101).

Khan and Masud (1963), a disciple of Winnicott, advances the notion of cumulative trauma based on "breaches in the mother's role as a protective shield" against excitations throughout the child's development. These breaches, he says, "cumulate silently and invisibly" (Khan and Masud, 1963, p. 47). Many intersubjectivists consider that traumatic situations are the product of early failed interactions between the baby and the needed objects (poor empathetic attunement, emotional exploitation), that is, of the lack of a modulating, supportive intersubjective context.

Early situations with potentially traumatic effects are not traumatic *per se*. They will only lead to illness if the environment cannot respond, a failure that will prevent these situations from becoming experience. If the environment does not provide holding and empathy to validate the pain of experience, the baby will lack adequate affective regulation, and its incipient self will suffer disorganization and disintegration (Shane and Shane, 1990). We cannot fail to mention the impact of present-day events (international terrorism, mass migrations) on our societies. Laurent (2004, p. 54) asserts: "All of us, minors or not, will increasingly be the children of real trauma," since today "what cannot be programmed becomes trauma."

6 Narcissistic disorders, severely ill patients
Psychotics and borderline personalities

Narcissism is a term that evokes an array of meanings in our discipline in relation both to the evolution of the psyche and to clinical work. As W. Baranger points out, "In psychoanalytic theorizing, the concept of narcissism occupies a position similar to that of identification: both led to a profound restructuring of psychoanalytic theory." "Narcissism," he adds, "completely overturned the theory of instincts" (W. Baranger, 1991, p. 108). The following list shows the different meanings of the term. I will dwell on those used by Winnicott and Kohut when discussing clinical work with severely ill patients.

I Narcissism and the vicissitudes of psychic development

I.a A developmental stage or phase situated between autoerotism and object love. It is a transitory stage, but it also corresponds to the consolidation of pregenital autoerotic dispersion. In 1914 Freud states that narcissism is "a new psychical action" (p. 77). This statement alludes to the convergence of scattered pregenital autoerotic zones into a totality that starts to be recognized as unique.

I.b Narcissistic object choice: In clinical practice, it leads to the absence of me/not-me differentiation. Freud (1914c) discusses this type of narcissistic choice in "On Narcissism: An Introduction." We should recall here that this choice involves an object that is identical to oneself, that is, like a part of oneself or is related to one's ideal (what one was or would like to be). There are numerous literary allusions to this type of choice. For instance, in *La magia de la niñez* (The Magic of Childhood) Gudbergur Bergsson (2004) claims that poets only draw from their own views and experiences, and everything that is outside themselves is just conjecture.

I.c Narcissistic identification ("He's a part of me" or "I'm a part of her"): Basic projective identification mechanisms described by Melanie Klein that erase subject/object differences and lead to the world of the One.

I.d Narcissism as a libidinal supplement of egotism.

II Narcissism in clinical practice

II.a Narcissistic features (pride, arrogance)

II.b Narcissistic injury (related to amour-propre, self-esteem)

II.c Narcissism of small differences, described by Freud

II.d Narcissism as a perversion (the body, or part of it, as a homosexual love object)

II.e Narcissistic resistances perceived during the treatment

It is worth remembering here other concepts that are useful for the development of a new clinical psychopathology:

- Good and bad (pathological) narcissism, or life narcissism and death narcissism, according to Green (2001). This author highlights a form of narcissism that is "in love with death" and that thwarts the formation of the psychic structure. Life narcissism, contrariwise, creates bonds that give rise to that structure.
- "Good" narcissism, according to Sandler and Joffe (1967, p. 63), is "an ideal state (...) which is fundamentally affective and which normally accompanies the harmonious and integrated functioning of all the biological and mental structures."
- Healthy narcissism entails an adequate or suitable measure of amour-propre, which varies in each life stage and is highest during adolescence. This good narcissism involves accurate and realistic representations of the self. Bad narcissism, instead, leads to self-centredness as a defence against pathological object bonds. In the psychoanalytic milieu, however, *narcissistic* still has a negative sense, and rarely refers to someone who has adequate self-esteem.

The above list does not encompass all the uses of this term,[1] which, like many classic concepts, has suffered a number of slippages in meaning. (The same has happened with transference, acting out, and perversion.) In clinical work, narcissism is a vast domain that ranges from fanatical thought, which leaves no room for others, to self-esteem disorders, to the blurring of the boundaries with one's fellow beings and the experience of (un)reality. Depersonalization, derealization, and estrangement disorders are the product of the loss of narcissistic values. These values help keep the sense of identity in place and generate a sense of emptiness in a crisis.

In previous chapters, I stated that narcissism constitutes a unique way of experiencing the object as part of the self. This bonding mode is closely tied to the appearance of self-esteem disorders. Based on narcissistic transferences, Kohut describes different disorders that affect subjects' personality and behaviour. He will later call these transferences "object transferences of the self," and will define the object as narcissistically charged. Subjects relate to this object in three different ways, namely, through mirror, idealizing, and alter ego transferences, which are indispensable for the child's survival and development. Children need to be mirrored and a figure (a selfobject) to idealize, and later an object that will operate as a peer (alter ego).

The appearance of one of these transference modes in the analysis is the consequence of deficiencies in subjects' relationship with their selfobjects. Deficits in patients' personality represent a halt in their psychic development. The latter may resume its course with new impetus (like Balint's new beginning) if the analyst responds empathically, in the manner of the needed selfobject. Patients need such an object as a bridge to continue to grow.[2]

I also stressed earlier that Kohut describes two types of self disorders, namely, primary disorders (psychosis, borderline personality disorders, and addiction) and secondary disorders (narcissistic personality disorders and neuroses). Let us look first at Narcissistic Personality Disorders (NPD), which display a particular type of transference that constitutes their most relevant sign. This type of transference will be gradually but firmly established insofar as the analyst responds empathically. Kohut et al. (2005) have described different narcissistic personalities. The one depicted by Kernberg (1979) corresponds to axis II, group B.[3]

According to Kohut, subjects who suffer from NPD experience a sense of fragility, of imminent fall that accompanies them during their entire development. They tend to go unnoticed and avoid being the centre of attention. They experienced object lack or deficit during their development, and are sensitive, shy, and easily wounded. We could say that, broadly speaking, there are two subtypes of NPDs, namely, vulnerable/sensitive and grandiose/exhibitionist. Yet the NPDs described by Kohut reach an acceptable level of social functioning, and if they are aggressive, it is when they suffer narcissistic injuries. The illnesses studied by Kernberg, instead, closely resemble borderline personality disorders. Patients suffering from these disorders are arrogant, aggressive, envious, and grandiose. Kohut considers that idealization in the transference is acceptable and constitutes a necessary attempt to enact a phase that was absent in childhood. According to Kernberg, contrariwise, idealization is always defensive in the face of negative feelings (anger, envy, contempt).

These postulations make it possible to link culture and the production of psychopathology. We can view the emergence of human suffering after World War II as a consequence of socio-historical change. Mental pain stems from social phenomena such as anonymity, the lack of availability of fellow beings, and the particular features of social interactions.

Winnicott was always reluctant to use the concept of narcissism. In 1966, he states as follows: "I have never been satisfied with the use of the word 'narcissistic' (...) because the whole concept of narcissism leaves out the tremendous differences that result from the general attitude and behaviour of the mother" (Winnicott, 1989, p. 191). He thus views primary narcissism as a state that appears during individuals' subjective bond with the object, when they experience the environment as part of their self.

Severely ill, psychotic, and borderline patients

When do we classify a patient as severely ill? We could draw from psychiatric manuals' description of symptoms that indicate severity. Yet the various psychoanalytic hypotheses concerning grave illness, which do not always converge, have enriched the debate on this topic. Based on a variety of frames of reference, we may consider that the following patients are severely ill:

– those who cannot distinguish between memory and transference (Freud, 1912);
– those who have been severely traumatized, described by Masud Khan,[4] Herbert Rosenfeld (1979), and Joyce McDougall (1980);
– those who have not been able to develop a transitional space (Winnicott, 1971);
– those who live only in the selfobject transference (Kohut, 1977);
– those who have not achieved a representability that protects them from terror (Botella, 1997).[5]

What other perspectives are there concerning the gravity of patients' illnesses? We can keep enumerating definitions. A seriously ill patient is the one who:

– lacks an observing ego as a psychic tool, a tool that enables subjects to take distance and is represented by the expression "as if";
– needs the therapist to worry about him or her;
– needs others as objects to satisfy needs rather than desires;
– needs a supportive network and demands that others perform this role;
– needs something more than the therapist's words; or
– did not mature at the right time and, therefore, is not healthy but "pseudo" or "over" adjusted.

Killingmo (1989) speaks about patients with a deficit pathology. When working with these patients, we should try to help them experience a sense of self. Or, as the author puts it, our aim is that patients will feel that something exists rather than that they find something they lost. These patients need affirmative interventions from the analyst to internalize object relations that had not been internalized earlier. This internalization will allow them to confirm the validity of their experience.

We could also think of severely ill patients as those who do not adjust to a preestablished setting. I have already referred to the original setting, which was designed for neurotic patients. If we try to "adapt" severely ill patients to the classic setting without taking their specific traits into account, they may appear to do extremely well, thanks to the false aspects of their self (they will obsessively comply with time and space rules, fees, and so on).

Some comments about borderline and psychotic patients

I will not describe the clinical aspects of borderline or psychotic personalities, categories that, albeit steadily expanding, start taking shape in the
1940s and may be easily found in present-day psychiatry books or in psychoanalytic literature. I will only summarize the ideas of authors who are
original in their approach.

a   Kernberg (1975, p. 3) stresses that borderline patients present with "a
    rather specific and remarkably stable form of pathological ego struc-
    ture" that involves a halt in development. They usually display the fol-
    lowing features:

    –   chronic diffuse anxiety;
    –   polysymptomatic neurosis;
    –   object instability and great dependence, with labile bonds and lack
        of constancy;
    –   specific affects (rage, panic) and primitive ego defences against
        these affects;
    –   intolerance to frustration and other expressions of ego weakness,
        for example, difficulty to synthesize and to pay attention;
    –   superficial adaptation to reality;
    –   polymorphous and sometimes perverse sexuality (e.g., sadomaso-
        chism); and
    –   multiple personality based on superficial identifications.

b   Grinker and others (1968) mention four basic characteristics:

    –   fury or anger affect;
    –   dependence and rigidity in emotional relationships;
    –   lack of consistent self-identity (they see themselves as playing a
        role); and
    –   empty depression.

c   According to Paz (1969), these are some of the features of borderline
    patients:

    –   they cannot distinguish impulses from affects and bodily sensations;
    –   they confuse past and present;
    –   they cannot postpone release (tendency toward impulsiveness); and
    –   they do not hallucinate or rave, but their judgement is disturbed.

d   Green (1975) accurately argues that the borderline state is a "borderline
    state of analyzability" (p. 30), and considers that "the implicit model
    of borderline states leads us back to the contradiction formed by the
    duality of separation anxiety/intrusion anxiety" (p. 40). This author de-
    scribes four extreme defences in these patients: somatic exclusion, ex-
    pulsion via action, splitting, and decathexis.

e   Kohut (1971) does not consider these patients analysable, and states that a patient may be borderline for one analyst and not for another, depending on the therapist's ability to establish an empathic bond.
f   Winnicott, as I mentioned earlier, considers that borderline patients are mainly psychotic subjects who have achieved neurotic defences.

We can define borderline patients as subjects who have deficit pathologies stemming from helplessness caused by failures in early development and have been able to establish "protective" neurotic defences. The notion of borderline personality evolved over time. Today, this illness is conceptualized (and hence treated) as a pathology that is closer to affective disorders than to schizophrenia. In these patients, frequent depressions are not connected with guilt; they are empty of affect – full of boredom. Only anger, as their major emotion, introduces some variety. Emerging as an outburst, it allows them to vent their peculiar anxiety of disintegration, which is expressed as an unbearable sense of emptiness.

Fiorini (1999, p. 211) offers an original conception about the current manifestation of this illness. "It is my impression," he states,

> that borderline phenomena (unlike the classic categories of neurosis, psychosis, and perversion, which entail certain predictable models or patterns) are chaotic; they adopt variable forms depending on the individual and on that individual's moments. Consequently, borderline patients appear to be much more complex, amidst a broad network of interactions.

And he adds:

> Prigogine says that the farther away an object or a system is from equilibrium (the greater its disequilibrium), the greater will be the influence it receives from elements in the environment. The borderline patient, characterized, precisely, by being far from equilibrium, is much more sensitive to all kinds of variables (...) [and] challenges the features of intrapsychic life.
>
> (ibid.)

Regarding psychoses, Winnicott (1967b) argues that "insanity is usually not a regression, which has an element of trust in it; it is rather a sophisticated arrangement of defenses whose object is to prevent a repetition of disintegration" (1986, p. 28). This author, therefore, values the setting provided by the psychiatrist, which mimics a holding environment that is specific for each patient and facilitates the recreation of hope, a concept related to health. In this article Winnicott asserts that severe mental illness is the result of a halt in development. Thus, when working with seriously ill patients, we must remove the obstacle impeding it. Individuals, then, will grow, thanks to "inherited tendencies that fiercely drive the individual on in a growth process" (ibid., p. 144).

In this sense, colleagues may find his simple taxonomy useful. This taxonomy divides patients into two categories. The first corresponds to those who received enough care during childhood and whose current suffering derives from classic conflicts. These patients' development disorders are deep. The second corresponds to those who suffered a deficit during their early care (early failure of the good-enough mother function). These patients present with early development disorders.

I mentioned before that Winnicott (1954) considers that borderline patients preserve a psychotic core. We should clarify here that for this author, psychosis involves a failure of environmental adaptation during the first developmental stages. Adaptation, in this case, refers to the supporting environment, which individuals cannot recognize as external to them – they are fused with it. For this reason, psychotic patients who are surrounded by a new environment may recover spontaneously, while psychoneurotic patients truly need the analyst.

Psychosis, according to Winnicott, is closely related to health. In psychotic subjects, innumerable situations of environmental failure have remained frozen and may be reached and thawed by a variety of healing phenomena that are part of everyday life, such as friendships or care received during a physical illness. Consequently, he believes that psychosis is associated with environmental failure during an early stage of emotional development. Feelings of futility and unreality are typical of the false self, which develops as a shield for the true self.

Notes

1　I left out the expression "narcissistic culture," which is used as a synonym for postmodernity ("culture of the image") and denotes superficiality and inconsistency.

2　See Borgogno (2005) for a comprehensive description of arrested development as it presents in clinical practice.

3　According to the DSM, the basic feature of a narcissistic personality disorder is a general pattern of grandiosity, a need to be admired, and a lack of empathy that start at the beginning of adulthood and occur in different contexts. Subjects are usually male and have a grandiose sense of self-importance. They tend to overvalue their abilities and exaggerate their knowledge and qualities, so they often strike others as boastful and conceited. They may easily accept the exaggerated value attributed to their acts by others and are surprised when they do not receive the praise they expect and believe they deserve. Subjects with a narcissistic disorder think they are superior, special, or unique, and expect others to recognize them as such. They think that they can only be understood by or relate to other special or high-status people, and attribute those who are close to them the qualities of "unique," "perfect," or "talented."

　　In general, they demand excessive admiration. Their self-esteem is almost always very fragile. They may be worried about doing things well enough and about others' opinion of them. Such concern tends to manifest itself as a constant need for attention and admiration; they are confused or angry if they do not receive continuous attention. For instance, they may assume they do not need to stand in line, and believe their priorities are so important that everyone must acquiesce to them. As a result, they become irritated if others do not help them with their work, which is "so important." This pretentiousness, accompanied by a lack of sensitivity toward others' wishes and needs, may lead to a conscious or unconscious exploitation of their fellow beings.

Generally speaking, subjects with a narcissistic personality disorder lack empathy and have a hard time recognizing the wishes, subjective experiences, and feelings of others. When they do, they will likely deride them as signs of weakness or vulnerability. Those who establish bonds with subjects with this type of disorder often develop emotional coldness and lack of interest toward them. Subjects with this disorder usually envy others or believe that others envy them. They may envy other people's success and possessions, as they believe that they are more deserving than those people of such achievements, admiration, or privileges. They frequently show a snobbish, derisory, or arrogant attitude.

4 Masud Khan (1973) considers that the mother's failure to protect the baby from excitations (in particular, from her own hatred toward it) during the preverbal stage of the mother-child relationship contributes to the child's trauma.

5 C. and S. Botella have thoroughly studied representations. Psychoanalysis starts from the theory of representation, which corresponds to the theory of the drives. The absence of the object may be equivalent "to the loss of its representation, the heir to hallucinatory wish-fulfilment, which is a synonym for distress" (Botella and Botella, 2005, p. 29). This situation would correspond to an initial psychic functioning with contradictory interests rather than to a classic conflict.

> The danger of the loss of representation (not of the object) provokes a real void with an implosive effect, precipitating the hated perception in the psyche (…) the small child who wakes up terrified, with a wild expression in his eyes, has only been able to preserve his investments of object-representations, his desire, thanks to the nightmare.
>
> (ibid., p. 30)

The fantasy threat of the nightmare ultimately works as a defence that prevents the loss of representation and, therefore, psychic death. With "non-represented" patients, analysts do not interpret a fantasy in the face of loss but provide the flooded ego with an image in order to fill the gap opened by the trauma and thus restore psychic continuity.

Stories form a bridge between child and adult that drives the disorganized experience toward representation. Trauma implies lack of representation (and an intense mobilization with great hallucinatory activity that feeds on the negativity of the original trace and restores a representation that has been transformed, transfigured into hallucination or perception). For these authors, traumatic neurosis is in itself a psychopathological model that is the opposite of psychoneurosis and is potentially always present in the psyche. What cannot be psychically worked through should be defined as traumatic. It is not a mere repetition of the experience of suffering. Rather, the ego participates actively, trying to render psychic (to mentalize) a surplus of energy, a negativity that, quoting Winnicott, is "what is not yet experienced [but] has nevertheless happened in the past" (Winnicott, 1974, p. 105).

7 Edition-Reedition

Some thoughts based on Winnicott's contributions to the understanding and treatment of psychosis and other severe pathologies[1]

In this chapter I develop the idea that only in a new bond can certain symptoms be resolved that emerged due to an intense, prolonged pathological relationship at the beginning of a person's life. In particular, I aim to show that it is through the mechanism that Lerner and I have called *edition* (Lerner and Nemirovsky, 1989, 1990, 1992), which differs from the traditional notion of transference repetition, that patients can perceive what they were unable to experience in the past and thus integrate it into the self. Guided by Winnicott's ideas, for example "We are poor indeed if we are only sane." (D. W. Winnicott, 1992 [1945], p. 150), I understand that a successful treatment of a severe illness requires that the patient meet with an object that enables the actualization of early unmet needs. These needs were frozen until a meeting might take place that would facilitate their emergence.

Some considerations about the diagnosis of psychosis

A comprehensive definition of psychosis, agreed upon among colleagues who have worked extensively with severely ill patients, should not leave out features such as severe disorganization of the personality and marked libidinal and ego regression, or phenomenological descriptions such as bizarre behaviour, delirious ideas, labile and intense emotional reactions, and certainly a significantly disturbed relationship with the real world. Hallucinations, obstacles to thought processes, and hypochondria are also prominent traits.

Kaplan and Sadock (1988, p. 170) have chosen three parameters that, in their view, are relevant to define psychoses: "inability to distinguish reality from fantasy; impaired reality testing, with creation of a new reality." If most elements summarized in these definitions are present in our prospective patient, we will have no doubt about the diagnosis. If, in addition, we find several of the symptoms outlined above, it is more than likely that the patient is belatedly seeking help and that the illness started several years earlier (and that he or she has had more than one therapeutic experience since its onset). For this reason, crystallized symptoms and restitution processes have configured so rigid a stereotyped picture that if several colleagues observed the patient, even if their theoretical perspectives differed, they would offer the same or a slightly different diagnosis.

It is unlikely that we will be able to achieve a cure after years of chronic disease. The analytic bond will face transferences that will generate permanent distortions and determine a stereotyped view that will only allow the therapist to direct his or her therapeutic efforts toward rehabilitation. We should recall here that Freud (1917–1919) complains thus about the Wolf-Man: "Personal peculiarities in the patient and a national character that was foreign to ours made the task of feeling one's way into his mind a laborious one." Then he adds:

> The contrast between the patient's agreeable and affable personality, his acute intelligence and his nice-mindedness on the one hand, and his completely unbridled instinctual life on the other, necessitated an excessively long process of preparatory education, and this made a general perspective more difficult.
>
> (Freud, 1918 [1914], p. 104)

We must admit that those patients whom we might generically call *severely ill* will require from us an especially careful, cautious, and neutral attitude (which I discussed earlier) in order to prevent adverse results. Such carefulness, which should accompany every intervention, derives from Winnicott's concept of treatment, and this concept inspired the ideas developed here. Winnicott examines the notion of regression in the context of the treatment of psychotic patients – more specifically, regression to their early dependence on their surrounding environment. Because of the "tendency towards a re-establishment of dependence," the environment must necessarily be taken into account. Such tendency to regression, he argues, is "part of the capacity of the individual to bring about self-cure," and "gives an indication from the patient to the analyst as to how the analyst should behave rather than how he should interpret."

Psychosis, therefore,

> is no longer to be ascribed to a reaction to anxiety associated with the Oedipus complex, or as a regression to a fixation point, or to be linked specifically with a position in the process of the individual's instinctual development. Instead it could be postulated that the regressive tendency in a psychotic case is part of the ill individual's communication, which the analyst can understand in the same way that he understands the hysterical symptom as a communication. The regression represents the psychotic individual's hope that certain aspects of the environment which failed originally may be relived, with the environment this time succeeding instead of failing in its function of facilitating the inherited tendency in the individual to develop and to mature.
>
> (Winnicott, 1959–1964, p. 128)

Even at the risk of being redundant, we should state once again that Winnicott (1971) speaks of borderline personalities as having a psychotic core and rigid defences. These patients, therefore, present with psychopathological and therapeutic problems similar to those of psychotics. That is why I included them in the group of severely ill patients. It is particularly, thanks to our work with them, that we gradually learn that taxonomical variations can only be diagnosed in the context of a bond. For this reason, creating an environment that generates the fewest possible negative reactions is essential. The diagnosis and, undoubtedly, the prognosis of the case will hence depend on the quality of this bond and, above all, on our attitude and behaviour.

When attributing a "bizarre behaviour" or certain "emotional reactions" to patients, we must not only take into account the cultural context (local codes) but also consider that our own attitude is a critical factor in the establishment of the psychological field and, therefore, in the emergence of certain behavioural specificities in the patient. Later on, the consensus we reach with our professional peers will enable us to choose the right diagnostic category. Still, we must always maintain a flexible, ever-evolving taxonomy so as to avoid rigidities that will impoverish our thinking. It is worth reiterating here that only a new bond that can repair the early damaged one may facilitate the resolution of pathological developments resulting from a failed early relationship.

A perspective on severe pathologies

Winnicott (1960, p. 141) clearly distinguishes early needs from instincts ("It must be emphasized that in referring to the meeting of infant needs I am not referring to the satisfaction of instincts"), and groups the former in three categories, namely, holding, handling, and object-presenting. These needs must produce specific actions from the environment (the earliest environment is the preoccupation of the maternal figure) so that human subjects can integrate, personalize, and access reality in their journey toward independence. It is based on his vast, heterogeneous experience with severely ill patients that Winnicott argues that if, due to a variety of situations, responses from an adequate, critical, and specific object are absent, early needs will remain frozen, waiting for a receptive, non-"reactive" context.

The model offered by Winnicott and his many followers, uncompromisingly focused on bonds, is scientifically grounded in Freudian and Kleinian developments. Yet our author, as well as many of his predecessors, shows two important differences with such developments. He distances himself from instinct-based, and hence deterministic, ideas, and prioritizes environmental factors in human upbringing. From this perspective, the environment constitutes an irreplaceable provider of objects that will satisfy needs, and later, desires.

If we explore the psychoanalytic literature, we will find that Winnicott was not alone in the essential aspects of his approach. We already pointed out similarities with Fairbairn (1941). It is also at this time that Bowlby (1940) writes his first paper on the influence of the environment in the development of neuroses. In the next decade, Balint (1957) develops his theory, based on what he calls the basic fault. More recently, the colleagues who accompanied Winnicott in the middle group and those whose ideas were close to his in the US expanded on some of his points of view. These authors were Mahler (1968), Erikson (1950), Searles (1965), Kohut (1966), and their followers.

We should now ask the following question: Why is it that four or five decades after the birth of psychoanalysis, many of these thinkers look at psychic phenomena from such different perspectives? Why do bonding approaches are in the foreground of contemporary psychoanalytic theory? What has happened to the traditional Oedipus complex? There are many factors that have led to this state of affairs (among them, innovators' personal background), but I would like to stress one element that seems essential to me. The development of an illness and the way we conceive of it also depend on the values that are prevalent at the time. During modernity (and we can confirm this with every Freudian paradigm), the search for knowledge and truth were the guiding star of every researcher – positive knowledge, and truth as the opposite of appearance and lies.

Regarding the value of the environment in the aetiology of psychosis, we should recall that our author states as follows: "Relaxation for an infant means not feeling a need to integrate, the mother's ego-supportive function being taken for granted" (Winnicott, 1960, p. 61). Integration is closely linked to the "supportive" environmental function in its material and/or metaphorical sense. Therefore, if we provide a setting that facilitates the creation of a "supportive" environment, which should probably be specific for each patient, we will enable patients to experience hope, as this insightful author points out, and we will certainly come closer to a glimpse of health. In this regard, Winnicott emphasizes the bond, a bond of presence and availability and, consequently, of hope. Don't these formulations help us elucidate the issues at stake in the treatment of severely ill patients?

The reedition/edition controversy: can we create what never was?

The Freudian concept of repetition

Freud writes in "Remembering, Repeating and Working Through":

> ...the patient (...) repeats everything that has already made its way from the sources of the repressed into his manifest personality – his inhibitions and unserviceable attitudes and his pathological character-traits. He also repeats all his symptoms in the course of the treatment.

And he adds:

> In drawing attention to the compulsion to repeat we have acquired no new fact but only a more comprehensive view. We have only made it clear to ourselves that the patient's state of being ill cannot cease with the beginning of his analysis, and that we must treat his illness, not as an event of the past, but as a present-day force. This state of illness is brought, piece by piece, within the field and range of operation of the treatment, and while the patient experiences it as something real and contemporary, we have to do our therapeutic work on it, which consists in a large measure in tracing it back to the past.
>
> (Freud, 1914, pp. 151–152)

Later, in the *Introductory Lectures to Psychoanalysis* (1916 [1917]), he insists on defining the transference relationship as repetition. That is why we often see our patients abandon their neurotic symptoms. The transference, which represents a camouflaged repetition of their old neurosis, will lead to changes in the expression of that neurosis. The positive consequence is that the key aspects of this pathology may be better grasped and elucidated, for the therapist has now reached its core. A new neurosis replaces the first one within the analyst/patient bond. Freud states in this regard: "the mastering of this new, artificial neurosis coincides with getting rid of the illness which was originally brought to the treatment – with the accomplishment of our therapeutic task" (Freud, 1916 [1917], p. 444).

Freud formulated a visionary question that he left unanswered:

> Nor can I think that it would be a disaster to the trend of our researches, if what lies before us is the discovery that in severe psychoses the ego-instincts themselves have gone astray as a primary fact. The future will give the answer....
>
> (ibid., p. 430)

We are in that future, and we can see that Freud's intuition is one of the most relevant ideas to be studied by the various authors from whose work I have drawn. "Ego-instincts themselves," which were then viewed as opposed to sex instincts and which require a "specific action" to be satisfied, are based on a concept that is very close but not identical to Winnicott's "ego instincts."

As this author states, ego instincts are needs that must necessarily find their specific object in order to achieve integration, personification, and re-alization. We find the same idea in Kohut (1971) when he discusses the first object relations, which facilitate the establishment of a cohesive, vital, and harmonious self. To reach this end, the incipient self must find objects that will mirror it and which it can idealize. Bowlby (1969) also agrees with these views when he describes attachment behaviours, and so does Balint (1968), who postulates the presence of primary love. Similar theoretical concepts are present in McDougall's (1985) clinical experience as well.

If at the beginning of a baby's life the person who must *hold* and *tolerate* it (the depository of its trust) repeatedly fails, the baby will have developmental deficits. If, contrariwise, this person is able to fulfil the maternal functions, the baby will *be* – it will feel real and creative and will be able to live in its own body and to remain the same over time. When these early indispensable objects fail to establish a reliable *holding*, the baby's needs freeze until they find a better chance of getting the response they seek in friendship, poetry, or psychoanalysis. If a pertinent meeting does not occur, a breach will be produced that will lead the mind, and later the false self, to take the place of the person ("being instead of") in order to avoid chaos. In the most severe cases, this process will eventually even give rise to the defensive construction of a delirium.

Simultaneously with the publication by Winnicott of such important articles as "Primitive Emotional Development" (1945) and "Psychosis and Child Care" (1952), Erikson (1950) describes the epigenetic stages of human development. He starts with "basic trust," which entails both feeling physically comfortable and experiencing the least possible amount of fear and uncertainty. If these requirements are met, the baby will be able to feel the same trust when undergoing new experiences. If this first stage constitutes a good experience, moreover, it will leave behind a feeling of hope.

Let us go deeper into Winnicott's ideas. According to this author, analysts wait until patients can "present the environmental factors in terms that allow for their interpretation as projections." If the case is well chosen, "this result comes from the patient's capacity for confidence, which is rediscovered in the reliability of the analyst and the professional setting." Analysts may have to wait a long time. When the case is not suitable for traditional psychoanalysis, "the reliability of the analyst is the most important factor (or more important than interpretations) because the patient did not experience such reliability in the maternal care of infancy" (Winnicott, 1960a, p. 38). To learn how to make use of objects' reliability, therefore, patients must find it in their analyst's behaviour "for the first time."

It is worth highlighting the following concepts in Winnicott's text:

a   *The notion of a badly chosen case for traditional psychoanalysis*: Without starting a debate on what constitutes traditional psychoanalysis, we should stress that if analysts consider creativity an important value, they must invent (probably reinvent) a unique mode of meeting for each person they treat. What is immutable, then, what is "traditional," is not our technique (as I mentioned above, there is no "traditional technique," not even in Freudian protocols). Rather, it is that aspect of the treatment that is connected with ethics; we should never manipulate our patients, and we should respect their values. "In psycho-analysis as we know it," Winnicott claims in the same essay, "there is no trauma that is outside the individual's omnipotence" (ibid., p. 36).

When Winnicott classifies his patients according to their psychopathology, he looks at the degree of organization of the self; the existence of something true in it and its potential to become evident; the "porosity" of the false self; and finally, and this is a very significant contribution, analysts' ability to operate with these patients as we do with neurotic patients, that is, based mainly on interpretive activity. If this is not possible, Winnicott suggests using management techniques in which the frame, the setting, becomes more significant, and advances different categories that may be used to classify patients. I discuss these categories in the next chapter.

b   *Reliability*: I already indicated how dear this concept is for Winnicott, and for Erikson as well. We should recall here that so-called predepressive patients could not experience trust with their first objects. Winnicott unequivocally states his position in 1954: "Psychotic illness is related to an environmental deficiency at an early stage of the emotional development of the individual (...) and (...) can only be relieved by specialized environmental provision interlocked with the patient's regression." To this end, "the provision of a setting that gives confidence" is essential (Winnicott, 1954, p. 23). As we progress in our discipline, especially in our research into the analysis of severely ill patients, we gradually approach (with more tools) the helplessness that Freud (1926) associated with the experience of newborns. Doubtless, in these times, due to the characteristics of urban social organization, the search for a fellow being is motivated by the need for a meeting (with an object that may satisfy basic needs) rather than by sexual desire.

c   *For the first time*: with this reference to an event that happens effectively for the first time in the analysis, Winnicott plunges into the question of edition. This is how Lerner and I describe this concept:

> During the analytic experience, a sequence of situations that had not been inscribed during childhood (due to the lack of an ego substratum to do so) must be edited. We can now observe transferences, which we call need transferences, that do not repeat "automatically." Rather, they only do so if the analyst's empathic attitude makes it possible for them to be edited and to unfold. They are not re-impressions; they exist in a potential space, waiting for an object that allows them to emerge by performing specific actions. For edition to be possible, analysts must develop professional attitudes that are specific to each patient: mirroring, providing coherence, signifying and discriminating emotions, understanding the sequence of the manifest material.
>
> (Lerner and Nemirovsky, 1990, p. 177)

Only if analysts provide a reliable setting by creating a suitable environment and being available to their patients will the latter be able to attempt to trust them. There is no worse nostalgia than longing for what never happened, says the Spanish singer Joaquín Sabina (1990). Therefore, we wonder, where can we find what has not been edited yet?

And the answer is, in an encounter with another human being. Humans are born with a disposition to trust – if we want to survive, that is our only option. We start in the opposite end of the notion of responsibility, which begins to develop once we appropriate experiences that inform us of what we are capable of doing to others. Responsibility is the smallest for newborns and the highest for its parents, to whom it surrenders.

If the baby is disappointed (materially and metaphorically), it will develop symptoms that are typical of dissociative disorders, which we see in patients presenting with depersonalization or panic as well as in borderline and psychotic patients. Yet if everything goes well, that is, if the baby finds environmental responses where it seeks them, if the object is where it "must" be and satisfies needs and then gradually fails (since in the case of patients who are in a state of need, we cannot fail if we want to remain analysts), the right conditions will be created for patients to edit.

Let us look at another statement by Winnicott (1954) that supplements the notions we have been discussing. In speaking of patients' acting out during the session, he describes a sequence that unfolds after an acting-out episode. In this context, he states that "anger belonging to the original environmental failure situation (...) is being felt perhaps for the first time" (Winnicott, 1954, p. 25). In other words, subjects will react here, for the first time, in a way they could not react in the past. They probably obeyed or submitted (to the analyst and to the formal aspects of the relationship), and their anger was postponed, frozen until it could unfold in a context that would ensure its containment and the ensuing reparatory behaviour.

What does edition contain? Those experiences that could not be appropriated because they could be encompassed and, therefore, did not belong to the patient. Early environmental failure creates the fear of recurrence, and this fear is a sign of the endurance of that failure. The fear experienced by the person who has already suffered a breakdown, as well as the fear of repetition actualized in the transference, will be the sole indicator that will guide us in our attempt at reparation, in which we engage from our analytic position. The transference mode will be the one that Balint (1968) describes as basic fault, Winnicott (1974) as the fear of breakdown, and Lerner and I (Lerner and Nemirovsky, 1990), as "need transference."[2]

d   *In their analyst's behaviour*: Analysts must certainly behave themselves with all their patients, as Winnicott puts it, but we should state from the outset that this is neither a technical recommendation nor an ethical principle. This notion is especially meaningful with early traumatized patients (McDougall, 1980), and derives from the concept of *good-enough mother*. In clinical practice, it means that if analysts are authentic, that is, sensitive, constant, consistent, devoted, and tolerant with their own anger, if they have the qualities of a good-enough mother, patients will be able to delegate in them their false self. In complex cases, analysts must be ready to wait. This is not just rhetoric; sometimes we must wait years without taking revenge, and must support the family as well. And not only the patient's family – Searles (1966) has dared to state clearly that we must primarily support our own family.

To become the analysts of psychotic patients, analysts must "behave themselves." Winnicott (1971) tells a male patient: "I am listening to a girl. I know perfectly well that you are a man but I am listening to a girl, and I am talking to a girl." Then he addresses his readers: "I wish to emphasize that this has nothing to do with homosexuality." After a pause, the patient says: "If I were to tell someone about this girl I would be called mad." And the analyst: "It was not that you told this to anyone; it is *I* who see the girl and hear a girl talking, when actually there is a man on my couch. The mad person is *myself*." The narrative continues: "The patient said that he now felt sane in a mad environment." And later: "... this man had to fit into her [his mother's] idea that her baby would be and was a girl" (Winnicott, 1971, pp. 73–74; author's emphasis).

If we imagine for a moment that Winnicott had not been who he was and had "fit into" a certain way of analysing, into a single perspective (like the patient into his mother's idea), what would he have interpreted? He might have said something like, "You wish me to assume your feminine part" or, perhaps, "You want to make me see that..." and so on. In short, he would have pointed to the wrong path or blamed the patient. This sequence might have been just right for a therapist who, abusing the notion of projective identification, was trying to behave himself ... with theory! This imaginary therapist would not have dared to "be a mad person."

If Winnicott had not developed his environmental failure theory, what would he have seen? And, what if the patient had been "labelled" (by way of a pseudo-interpretation) as a homosexual? We could keep asking questions, but Winnicott offers us a model that eliminates spurious queries and advances other perspectives and motives that must be investigated. At this stage, a clarification is necessary: intense and constant disturbance in the satisfaction of the self's needs, always basic needs, generates the conditions for the psychotic illness to develop. Like my predecessors, however, I am not ruling out biochemical or genetic factors. Each of us contributes to the discussion from the knowledge he or she has acquired. What is left is the still-incipient task of integrating the various vertices of knowledge.

Some conclusions

To analyse psychotic patients, analysts must meet certain requirements: be bold, allow ourselves to be contradictory ... even dare to see the patient as the most important thing in our lives at this time, and later be able to leave all this behind. In this sense, the paths we take in the treatment of psychotic patients are idiosyncratic and demand great effort on our part to travel them, as well as the support of our own family. Family members will probably be affected, whether we like it or not, by unexpected calls from the patient if not by visits to our home or other ways of approaching us with a variety of messages.

What qualities must analysts have to treat psychotic patients? Mostly, they must tolerate being "non-existent" for long periods of time. If they pass the test, they will have to bear these patients' intense, changing, and usually acted-out transference. Moreover, they must be prepared to accept a spontaneous cure, something that does not happen with neurotic patients, who need the analyst's interpretive work. We should recall here my earlier quote from Winnicott (1954): "psychosis is closely related to health, in which innumerable environmental failure situations are frozen but are reached and unfrozen by the various healing phenomena of ordinary life, namely friendships, nursing during physical illness, poetry, etc., etc." (1954, p. 22).

Therapists must *be* and, starting from there, *do*. If they are not authentic, if their work is not embodied in their personality, they will not be in charge of the treatment for long; they will be rapidly reviled by patients with a deficit pathology, whose refined sensitivity always allows them to grasp more than analysts want to show. Perhaps patients will adjust (which would be more painful) to the little they may receive, and their history, the history of their illness will recur. Analysts who treat psychoses will treat one, two at a time at the most. They will not bear many more than that because for a long time, in order to survive, they will have to be a good-enough mother, no more, no less, and try to understand while avoiding explanations.

What are the limits of our understanding capacity as analysts?

> The following are specifically analytic tasks: mirroring; providing consistency; giving meaning to and discriminating emotions; understanding the sequence of the manifest material, and neither rejecting it as lacking value nor attributing value to it as a vehicle used by the unconscious to emerge; setting boundaries ("That's not good for you...") or giving suggestions ("Better postpone that decision for later") (Gioia, 1989); being patient, and being able to refrain from interpreting everything we perceive; allowing the patient to have intimacy with himself or herself; and being, at times, mute witnesses to our own exclusion.
>
> (Lerner and Nemirovsky, 1989, p. 102)

Patience is certainly an analytic feature, a primary resource, but to what extent must we practice it? "The boundaries of our attitude and our setting are not those of theory but those of empathy, patience, and the ability to continue to think. We can be that flexible without introducing parameters" (Lerner and Nemirovsky, 1990, p. 179). Waiting for patients to be able to own their anger is one of the hardest functions to be performed by the analyst of psychotic patients. It is comparable, perhaps, to tolerating the idealizing transference.

I am also talking about boldness; we must have the boldness to create and recreate exits, paths, and slants that will only materialize in this relationship. One of the examples is the case cited earlier, where Winnicott could renege, even if partially and temporarily, of his perception and tell a patient, "I see a man but I'm listening to a girl." Another important condition we must meet in order to analyse psychotic patients is feeling able to embrace the possibility of helping this particular patient by "living with" him or her for a while.

And what about the analyst's responsibility regarding analysands' reactions? When and how do we enable development (within a suitable environment), and when and how do we provoke reactions? Galli (1982) poses a very interesting question: Why is it that young therapists are more effective than more experienced ones in the treatment of psychotic patients? This author offers a tentative answer based on the fact that young people accept challenges to their role and knowledge more easily. We can think further in this direction, and argue that young people will likely cling less to theories that only allow them to look at clinical experience through a narrow gap. They also devote more time to each patient and, if their psychic health allows it, their viewpoint will be closer to common sense than to theory.

Last, I would like to ask a question and leave it unanswered so as to promote debate: Does the problem posed by psychotic patients lie in the types of transferences they develop, or do analysts have a hard time accepting these patients' odd mode of relating – distressing, challenging, demanding, and even ... maddening?

Notes

1 This chapter is a revised version of an article published in *Aperturas*, 3, November 1999.
2 In borderline patients, unmet and unprecedented needs persist and strive to find a satisfying object, and thus recur time and time again in the analytic bond. These needs will not always be rooted in the vicissitudes of the sex instincts. At the same time, the psychic structure cannot adequately process them. My clinical work has shown the validity of the following thesis: those transferences that we call need transferences, whose role is similar to the role of Freud's self-conservation instincts, require a suitable environment to emerge and be acknowledged in the bond. Such acknowledgment, moreover, will facilitate psychological development. Besides the well-known neurotic and psychotic transferences, Lerner and I propose the existence of a third transference that we call need transference. It is overriding and sometimes silent, but it is always present in those who have not been able to configure a tripartite structure (Gedo and Goldberg, 1980). When this transference dominates, interpreting it is useless and may even be harmful (Valeros, personal communication). Winnicott (1971) states as follows:

Interpretations, however accurate and well-timed, cannot provide the whole answer. In this particular part of the therapist's work interpretations are more of the nature of verbalization of experiences in the immediate present of the consultation experience, and the concept of an interpretation as a verbalization of the nascent conscious does not exactly apply here.

(Winnicott, 1971, p. 161)

What is repeated in this type of transference? Instinct is experienced as foreign, since an incipient or poorly developed self cannot appropriate it. There is no object contingency for reedited needs; the object must be specific. There is no frustration; either the need is satisfied or it is frozen and must wait for an opportunity to develop. Borderline patients' labile repression will not affect it, and dissociation may displace it from the transference field.

8 The setting and interpretation

Some thoughts on Winnicott's concepts[1]

Introduction: choosing the treatment according to the psychopathology

I will now go back to some of the concepts discussed in Chapter 5. My work with complicated patients (who are sometimes called severely ill or hard to access and are increasingly present in today's clinical practice) has led me to delve deeper into the work of certain authors (Ferenczi, Fairbairn, Kohut, Green, Kernberg, and McDougall, and especially Winnicott). I tried to establish a dialogue with these authors in order to develop a personal answer that would allow me to solve some theoretical problems and, even more so, some clinical questions. The source of the questions that guide our research is never simple. These questions are based on patients' contributions, which are always enigmatic. Therapists embark, along with our patients, on a journey toward the unknown, a journey full of intertwinements of different dimensions in the manner of our own complemental series. Personal histories, professional models, epochal and ideological variables, and political-institutional vicissitudes will combine to suggest ways of perceiving the transference and will determine complex direct and indirect countertransferences.[2]

We have a pressing need for conceptualizations that address the new clinical phenomena we are witnessing in our consulting rooms today. We have to learn from our practice, which differs from the work of past decades, and adapt our concepts so that we can think and operate with subjects who, half-perplexed, half-distressed, perceive themselves as "remote from everything" or "unreal," as I described earlier. We need new strategies to respond to their anxieties and, at the same time, we must develop theoretical concepts that will explain phenomena as ineffable and common as the ones that constitute patients' presenting problems today. In Wallerstein's (1988) terms, we need "clinical theories." In this sense, in his thorough approach to patients whose self shows different structural disorders, Kohut speaks of theories of a "comparatively low-level, i.e., comparatively experience-near, psychoanalytic abstraction" (Kohut, 1971, p. xv). We also need operational metapsychologies, such as Zukerfeld and Zonis Zukerfeld's (1999) metapsychology or Bleichmar's (1997) Modular-Transformational Approach to complex systems.[3]

Despite these efforts, the question I formulated still stands. Is any of the known metapsychologies broad enough to address everything we see in our practice today without forcing observable data or reducing their phenomenological richness? We must also look outside our customary field of exploration and engage in a more honest and openly transdisciplinary dialogue with other mental health disciplines, such as cognitive psychology and contemporary psychiatry, and with aetiology as well.

Our metapsychologies are based on the study of psychopathological organizations that are a product of their sociocultural context and that develop, above all, on the "edges" of categories. That is why borderline disorders have emerged on the boundary between psychosis and neurosis. Moreover, they are in constant expansion and now include subcategories that are not easily distinguishable from certain psychopathies, ambulatory schizophrenias, and the new range of "severe neuroses," such as obsessive compulsive or panic disorders, which are appearing in our consulting rooms with unprecedented frequency. It is likely that the impact of our current way of life on the structuring of psychopathology and practitioners' new ways of seeing make the taxonomy of pathological conditions increasingly complex.

Our need to classify is never fully satisfied, as shown by the various well-intentioned lists of the DSM, the ICD, and other taxonomical codes. These codes fail to encompass the very different expressions of psychic malaise in their diverse cultural definitions. Such expressions, which enhance clinical complexity, depend on the historical juncture, as do our professional work and the theories that support it. Our treatment cannot be "standard"; we must tailor it to each patient, acknowledging that each meeting is unique, just as each patient is. We could cling to modes of reasoning that would lead us to think that everything has already been said about the shape taken by our encounters with patients. Yet the custom-made nature of clinical work prevents us from settling into this reassuring belief, and so does our intuition that to build the bridge that will make treatment possible, we must follow a more complex path than the one we were shown in our training institutes.

As Winnicott said, "In the work I am describing [with patients whose early needs were not adequately satisfied] the setting becomes more important than the interpretation" (Winnicott, 1975 [1955–1956], p. 297), and in this way, he polarizes the terms setting/interpretation, while other authors believe that the setting tends to remain mute so that interpretations may take centre stage as the major figure of psychoanalytic activity. Since Ferenczi's early questioning (from 1919 on), which drove him to develop an active technique and hence to part ways with Freud, different authors have alluded to these difficult situations. They have called severely ill patients "severely traumatized" (McDougall, 1980), "non-represented" (Botella and Botella, 1997), or "traumatized" (H. Rosenfeld, 1965). Leclaire (1977) and Pontalis (1990) have also warned analysts about the abuse of interpretation.

In this context, I think we need to dwell on the early/deep dialectic, which is very useful in clinical practice. It is obvious that the psychoanalytic method proposes a journey backward aiming to reach those events that are closest to the birth of the psyche according to each school. In this way, each perspective builds its own "baby," whose last name corresponds to the school that gave birth to it. These babies (Freudian, Kleinian, Lacanian, Winnicottian, and so on) are not identical; they resemble each other as siblings do, but also present irreducible traits.

Pine (1990) points to convergences and divergences between the four psychologies, namely, drive, ego, object relations, and self psychologies. I already mentioned that Winnicott (1957) distinguishes between deep and early contents. The latter, which are not part of the self, make it possible for subjects' history to begin. I am referring to the support and presence provided by the environment during the first moments of extrauterine life. Early experiences offer a supporting net that enables content to acquire a certain shape. It would be useful to debate about the isomorphism between the early/deep and the context/text and container/contained pairs (while taking into account the different frames of reference underlying each of these pairs).

Slowly, what will later become deep is established as the content of the self. It derives from experience and is configured as internal world. Operating with the notion of *early* in mind involves recognizing the existence of dependence (on primary objects), as Freud points out in "Inhibitions, Symptom and Anxiety" (1926, p. 137): "It is the absence of the mother that is now the danger." Winnicott, in turn, takes up again the consequences of prematuration (the danger indicated by Freud) as "early situations," which start with the initial lack of differentiation between subject and environment and require "specific actions" (in Freudian terms) from the environment to meet the baby's needs.

Without fear of being wrong, we could equate these needs experienced by Winnicott's baby, which do not originate in the sex drive, with Freud's self-preservation drives. Winnicott considers that the environment provides not only food and warmth but also a real and metaphorical holding for the baby, as well as the ability to be handled by a fellow being as a specific action and to avail itself of the objects that surround it. Later, thanks to these solidly laid early foundations, affects and instincts tied to depressive phenomena and to hatred will gradually grant depth to the psyche. Early foundations support and justify the presence of depth; they act, let us say it once again, as a safety net for the contents that are deposited in the psyche, and thus the boundaries of the self are delineated.

Setting and process

The behaviour of the analyst, represented by what I have called the setting, by being good enough in the matter of adaptation to need, is gradually perceived by the patient as something that raises a hope that the true self may at last be able to take the risks involved in its starting to experience living.

D. Winnicott (1975 [1955–1956], p. 297)

The above refers to the developmental aspects of psychoanalytic theory, but also involves psychopathological concepts and technical conceptualizations resulting from these aspects. I will take these as a pretext to develop a variety of notions that will help clarify Winnicott's ideas on the setting and the professional's attitude as well as stress their usefulness in today's practice. I aim to analyse these quotes in detail, as they look simple but, faithful to the author's style, evoke complex ideas. I already discussed the abused notion of the good-enough mother, which has often been taken as a moral precept or as a basis to produce recommendations for motherly behaviour (or has been interpreted, rather maliciously, by those who have not even read Winnicott's work as a call for mothers to be kind).

We should also recall here that a good-enough mother plays a twofold role, simultaneously real and metaphorical; she must be continuously present. Today we would add to the features enumerated earlier the quality of *resilience*, defined as "the human capacity to face, overcome, and be strengthened or transformed by experiences of adversity" (Grotberg, qtd in Zukerfeld, 2002, p. 148). I argued previously that Winnicott's clinical psychopathology starts from these ideas and goes on to establish a distinction between two types of patients. These can be broadly defined as (a) those who have had enough care and whose needs have been sufficiently met, whose current suffering derives from deep conflicts (emotional conflicts, in terms of Oedipal guilt and ambivalence); and (b) those who have not been so fortunate and have suffered a repeated deficit of early care due to environmental failure.

The previous year, based on the "technical equipment they require of the analyst" (Winnicott, 1954, p. 16), Winnicott added a third category. Schematically, patients can be grouped as follows:

1 Neurotics or whole people (Winnicott, 1960b): This is the model of the personality that Freud used as a basis for his theories. These patients suffer due to conflicts at the level of interpersonal relations (jealousy, rivalry, guilt). They can distinguish between subject and object, me and not-me. Their basic defence is repression (usually successful). Love and hate are differentiated, which enables the development of a clear therapeutic alliance. In "The Importance of the Setting in Meeting Regression in Psycho-Analysis" (1964), Winnicott points out that in these cases, which he calls ordinary, "one is cashing in on the work done by the parents, and particularly by the mother, in the early childhood and infancy of the patient" (1989 [1964], pp. 96–97).

2 Depressives: This is the model Klein and post-Kleinian analysts used as a basis for their theory. According to Winnicott, these patients could not overcome the stage of concern, for they were unable to work through the guilt generated by destructive fantasies (if they love, they destroy), and thus live in constant dependence. Therefore, it is critical to address their state of mind. Their basic defences are failed repression,

splitting, and superficial (non-structural) identifications. From a clinical perspective, they are schizoid, borderline (nearer to neurosis), and melancholy.

3   Pre-depressives: This is the model that Winnicott used (as did Ferenczi, Balint, Searles, Green, and McDougall), although not exclusively, as a basis for his theories. These patients are unable to distinguish between inside and outside. There is no notion of alterity or of projective space. If the analyst "behaves himself," these patients' transference will enable the edition of the environment-mother function. The transference is basically fusional and based on needs. The right behaviour on the part of the analyst will allow patients to experience the first phases of psychic development in the analysis. Clinically, this group includes the most severe borderline disorders and psychosis. As I mentioned in the previous chapter, Winnicott refers to the treatment of these patients as "management," although in other works he speaks about psychoanalysis (1964).

I believe that when analysts choose management as a therapeutic strategy to create the basic conditions that will enable patients to reflect and play, they can only do so based on a psychoanalytic frame of reference. Faced with a pre-depressive patient, a psychiatrist with no psychoanalytic training will likely medicate or contain the patient and offer no expectations for the future. The analyst, contrariwise, will adopt an analytic attitude in the framework of the treatment and will thus promote patients' ability to integrate by establishing contact with them. Patients will be able to use their analyst's failures to grow as long as the analyst adapts to their needs. If analysts repeatedly prove their trustworthiness, they will be able to react with objective anger (which, under these circumstances, will take the place of Klein's negative transference).

In 1954, Winnicott states that "the whole set-up of psychoanalysis is a big reassurance, especially the reliable objectivity and behaviour of the analyst" (Winnicott, 1954, p. 24). In this opportunity, he mentions Bettelheim's (1967) concept of "empty fortress" when pointing out that the main task of the analyst is to offer a specialized set-up.[4] In the same article, Winnicott refers to "Freud's clinical setting." This is how he describes it:

> 1. At a stated time daily, five or six times a week, Freud put himself at the service of the patient. (This time was arranged to suit the convenience of both the analyst and the patient.) 2. The analyst would be reliably there, on time, alive, breathing.

Winnicott goes on to say that the analyst expressed both love and hate toward the patient – love, through his positive interest, hate, through the strict maintenance of a schedule and through the demand of fees – and that he expressed both openly.

4 The aim of the analysis would be to get into touch with the process of the patient, to understand the material presented, to communicate this understanding in words. Resistance implied suffering and could be allayed by interpretation.

5 The analyst's method was one of objective observation.

6 This work was to be done in a room, not a passage, a room that was quiet and not liable to sudden unpredictable sounds, yet not dead quiet and not free from ordinary house noises. This room would be lit properly, but not by a light staring in the face, and not by a variable light. The room would certainly not be dark and it would be comfortably warm. The patient would be lying on a couch, that is to say, comfortable, and probably a rug and some water would be available.

Next, Winnicott refers to the analyst's abstention from moral judgement. The analyst does not invade the space of the patient with information about his or her own life and ideas, and does not side with persecutory systems, even if these appear as actual situations that are shared with the patient.

7 In the analytic situation the analyst is much more reliable than people are in ordinary life – on the whole punctual, free from temper tantrums, free from compulsive falling in love, etc.

8 There is a very clear distinction in the analysis between fact and fantasy, so that the analyst is not hurt by an aggressive dream.

9 An absence of the talion reaction can be counted on.

10 The analyst survives (Winnicott, 1954, p. 22).

Winnicott's reading of the Freudian frame highlights his conception of the setting, which acquires great significance as a therapeutic tool. The illusory objectivity that would be obtained by establishing certain fixed variables moves to the background. It should be reiterated here that the stability inherent in the frame does not result from establishing rigid formal parameters but is synonymous with adequate reliability and emotion.

What can be measured as a quantity (time, space, and fees, among others) can be changed; it may even become unstable or shift without jeopardizing analytic work, as long as the analyst's reliability is preserved. We often verify this formulation when, during regressive periods in their treatment, patients are affected by our moving our office, raising our fees, or cancelling an appointment, but thanks to the containment of the reliably stable relationship with us, they react only minimally. Bleger (2012) refers to these situations extensively and views the setting as the depositary of psychotic or indiscriminate aspects of the personality. Usually silent, these aspects burst in when the setting is modified. Such irruptions, in my view, are associated with trust variables and the constancy of the bond, as I mentioned earlier, rather than with the setting in its temporal and spatial dimensions.

Turning back to Winnicott's ideas, I would like to underscore once again that the setting is established, maintained, and observed with the goal of facilitating patients' trust in the method and in the professional who is implementing it. Consequently, the setting is not an empty shell; temporal-spatial constants will allow professionals to display their analytic attitude (in Winnicott's terms, "to behave themselves"), which will enable them to find the specific action that meets each patient's needs. Analysts' attitude is decisive (and must be taken into account when making a referral or choosing an analyst, especially with very complicated patients). They must be able to keep calm and understand or empathize with the patient. We should not prioritize such features as knowledge or intelligence. Briefly, we should look for analysts who will be available and thus promote patients' ability to reflect.

Among the features that characterize the analytic attitude, we should include the calming role of para-verbal and preverbal components of our messages, which, acting as a framework for words, allow us to convey signs of recognition, reassurance, mirroring, holding, and attention that are all the more significant the greater the regression we encounter.[5] That is how Balint (1968) describes the analytic attitude when he discusses the notion of basic failure, and so do Bowlby, Stern, Emde, Lebovici, and others. In the same line, Loewald (1976) claims that we use language both to convey meaning and clarify situations, and to evoke mental states – to generate and link fields of experience.

For this author, language is a critical factor in the development of an original "primal density" in which feelings, perceptions, the others, and the self are all part of an indivisible unit. He argues that the preverbal field does not exist; language is an intrinsic dimension of human experience since birth. At the same time, in her review of Mitchell's posthumous book, Levinton (2001) points out that Beebe, Lachman, and Jaffe consider that babies are clearly capable of distinguishing slight differences in rhythm and inflection, frequency variation, and phonetic components of speech. At the beginning, says Loewald, words, the body, affects, and the relational connection are undifferentiated components of a unified experience.

Going back to Winnicott (1960b) and the notion of early needs, we could say that these are clearly differentiated from instinctive acts: "It must be emphasized that in referring to the meeting of infant needs I am not referring to the satisfaction of instincts" (1960b, p. 141). The environment (represented by the maternal figure described above) responds to the baby's needs with specific actions grouped in three categories, namely, holding, handling, and object-presenting. In 1954, our author argues that "with the regressed patient the word wish is incorrect; instead we use the word *need*" (Winnicott, 1954, p. 23; author's emphasis).

These needs are specific to each individual but go through a universal circuit. They include having one's needs guessed by the mother (cold? hunger?); being held "from the bottom" after birth; being mirrored in the mother's eyes, which gives the baby back its being; being important to one's parents; and many others. We should not be surprised by the fact that therapeutic meetings are original (unique or privileged) in a person's life. Are there reasons to think of patients as people who have enjoyed an infancy surrounded by objects that responded to their basic needs and who could hence edit a healthy environment?

When treating adults with early disorders, only very rarely are we not compelled to modify "traditional" setting parameters at some point during the treatment. Such modifications may go unnoticed; the setting does not necessarily speak loudly. For this reason, observing our own behaviour as analysts is very useful. We make slight changes: we adjust the light in the office for a certain patient; we offer more (or less) minutes in a particular session; we move or, contrariwise, never touch certain objects in the office, or make sure we do not change the tone of voice when addressing her. Or, we are certain that we must not interrupt a patient because we feel, due to a somewhat vague concern, that he will not tolerate our intervention, which may lead to a breakdown, even if we have something important to say.

To these examples, we should add situations with which we insistently fantasize and that sometimes, although probably seldom, materialize in needed actions, such as calling the patient's family, partner, or internist. Or, we may experience a sense of uncertainty at the end of the last (and sometimes only!) session of the week or prior to the holidays in view of the imminent separation, and may think (and sometimes say), "I'll leave you my phone/a colleague's phone/an email address where you can reach me during the holidays [as I myself have done] in case you need to get in touch with me." In short, different threads are needed to weave a safety net. At times, we have the fantasy of medicating the patient or of suggesting medication, especially if we are going to be away for some time.[6]

I call attention on these particular situations we go through, sometimes imperceptibly, when treating severely ill people so that practitioners will "make conscious" the need to establish a specific setting for each patient. To do so, we must take into account variables that go beyond our calendar. If we know how to interpret these situations, which stem from patients' primitive needs and are often imposed on us over the course of a treatment, we will be able to create a space that will foster patients' ability to reflect based on their use of us.

Some considerations about interpretation

Both Winnicott and Kohut trust that, as long as the atmosphere surrounding the infant is not "unhealthy" from the start, a healthy development will unfold. They do not point to a specific traumatic "fact" but to steady, constantly present pathologies in the environment surrounding the baby during its development. Rather than in a "great trauma," they are interested in the presence of a sordid, chronic atmosphere that will push the baby toward pathological development. The analytic setting can recreate or rectify this atmosphere, thereby becoming either an instrument that facilitates the recurrence of the traumatic atmosphere or a significant curative resource.

Kohut considers that interpretations should always be made in accordance with the environment and with patients' capacity to tolerate frustration so that they can provide an "optimal frustration." For this author, frustration is related to understanding. In the best-case scenario, analysts will understand their patients and recognize their legitimate concerns but will not enact them. It is an optimal frustration because the analyst's communication adapts to the patient's needs, thus strengthening the empathic connection.

Since Winnicott, the setting as a therapeutic tool, isomorphic with the human environment, has become particularly significant in patients who have suffered early traumas, usually categorized as depressive or pre-depressive. It is when tackling these psychopathological categories that analysts set aside Freud's aim to make conscious the unconscious. Winnicott (1971) alerts us to the danger of formulating interpretations without taking into consideration the degree of health or maturity reached by the patient. Interpretations must fit patients' developmental level and keep in mind the degree of regression they are undergoing at that moment of the treatment. If interpretations are offered when patients lack the ability to play, they provoke, at best, confusion and at worst, compliance or indoctrination.

It is at this time in our treatment of non-neurotic patients, when we see more darkness than light, that Winnicott's experience is useful and reassuring:

> ...it is only in recent years that I have become able to wait and wait for the natural evolution of the transference arising out of the patient's growing trust in the psychoanalytic technique and setting, and to avoid breaking up this natural process by making interpretations (...) It appals me to think how much deep change I have prevented or delayed in patients *in a certain classification category* [he is referring to borderline, schizoid, and severely ill patients] by my personal need to interpret. If only we can wait, the patient arrives at understanding creatively and with immense joy, and I now enjoy this joy more than I used to enjoy the sense of having been clever.
>
> (Winnicott, 1971, pp. 86–87)

And he states later that in patients

> who have a restricted capacity for introjective or projective identifying (...) interpretations are more of the nature of verbalization of experiences in the immediate present in the consultation experience, and the concept of an interpretation as a verbalization of the nascent conscious does not exactly apply here.
>
> (ibid., p. 161)

Jordán (2010) brilliantly describes analysts' participation in an object relation with the patient and, when the process is more advanced, how analysts enable patients to "use" them and the intersubjective relationship at play in the field of the bond. Interpretation also plays a role that we might call realistic, since analysts show both to what extent they are capable of receiving patients' communications and the limitations of their ability to understand. Patients will gradually recover their capacity to play, which is always at risk of being suppressed by a therapist who "knows too much."

Let us see how an experienced analyst such as H. Rosenfeld (1979) proceeds with a severely ill patient. This author offers some conclusions he reached after tackling a situation of impasse with a patient that was triggered by a delirious transference that found no response. He advises analysts to interpret very little and listen carefully to their patients' complaints. In particular, he warns, we should avoid interpreting projections or projective identifications in the transference, no matter how obvious their presence in the clinical material. Rather than interpreting, analysts should ask clarifying questions. Furthermore, in the case of acute and lasting transference psychoses, when patients want to sit and talk to the analyst face to face, the analyst should satisfy this need.

Rosenfeld suggests that analysts make technical choices that push interpretation to the background when they are trying to focus on patients' needs, which thaw at this time (as Etchegoyen does in the example below). Such needs cannot be set aside for the sake of "deep interpretations." As Rosenfeld argues, patients will then criticize analysts for not understanding what is happening to them, and they will likely be right. That is how these patients verbalize their demands (based on needs), which, provided that analysts' attitude is reliable, will strive to come out in order to produce (and now they do!) the desired response. Winnicott might say that interpretations are squiggles that must be created jointly by both participants.

A clinical exercise and some conclusions

Concerning the analytic attitude, Etchegoyen (1999) argues that there are "two ways (...) of understanding the setting: as a behavioural event or as a mental attitude" (Etchegoyen, 1999, p. 523). Naturally, this author leaves out the "ritual" aspect of behaviour and suggests that the setting is largely the result of the analyst's mental attitude. He then vividly illustrates these ideas with clinical examples. Among them, he recounts the story of a patient who had had orthopaedic surgery and had a very hard time walking and lying down. Right after the surgery, she called Etchegoyen and asked if he could put some extra cushions on the couch so that she wouldn't miss so many sessions, and seemed willing to accept his decision.

> The next day she came to the consulting room accompanied by a nurse, and Etchegoyen decided to lead her by the arm himself to the consulting room and helped her to make herself comfortable on the couch. He preferred to lead her by the arm himself into the consulting room, despite the physical contact this implied; to delegate this to the nurse would have been inconsistent with his setting, since no person other than his patient ever entered his consulting-room.

Then he refers to the example as follows: "It is evident that this decision is very debatable, and if another analyst had decided to do the opposite, I would never think him mistaken" (Etchegoyen, 1999, p. 524).

This experienced analyst decided not to let the nurse accompany the patient into his consulting room, despite the fact that this decision involved physical contact. What led him to adopt this very kind and thoughtful, although risky, attitude? Aiming to examine these concepts and to clarify different viewpoints, I would like to hypothesize that the analyst may have perceived this patient's needs and, in doing so, facilitated their unfolding in the analysis. From my perspective, these are needs related to early problems, that is, the need for real and metaphorical holding and handling, and probably to all those needs that coexist mutely in every human contact. Winnicott would say that they are frozen, waiting for the time when they can be brought into play, that is, for a reliable environment.

The environment created in this case, probably triggered by the analyst's emotional commotion at the patient's condition, shows that the analyst is available, sensitive, and vulnerable. These traits are all present in Winnicott's figure of the good-enough mother [which recalls Hartmann's (1939) notion of "average expectable environment"]. Such "common sense," innocent gestures allow us to establish a human contact that makes communication possible. I am not referring to the physical aspects of contact but to a relationship that facilitates a trusting connection between two people. An asymmetrical bond like the analyst-patient relationship allows the recreation (or, more likely, the creation) of an environment that will make it possible to return to those marks left by early failures, failures that led to withdrawal where there should have been contact.

The experienced analyst's attitude reproduces the environment recreated by Winnicott with one of his patients in *Playing and Reality* (1971). This environment is represented by the metaphor of the oil that makes gears run smoothly or by the idea Kohut (1979) conveys so well when he states that its surroundings are as necessary to the infant as oxygen is to breathing. These environmental objects (the environment mother is different from the mother as an object of the drive, a conceptual difference upon which Winnicott insists) can facilitate the baby's development, and will later play a role in the positive transference described by Freud. It goes without saying that these objects are part of the life history of the patients analysed by Freud or, better yet, of the psychic material that Freud analyses in these patients, but they are rarely contemplated in his medical histories or in the medical histories of later authors.

In "Further Remarks on the Theory of the Parent-Infant Relationship" (1989 [1961]) Winnicott states:

> In the psychoanalysis of a case well chosen for classical analysis the clinical distress comes in the form of anxiety, associated with memories and dreams and phantasies. But as analysts we get involved in the

treatment of patients whose *actual clinical breakdowns of infancy* must be remembered by being re-lived in the transference. In all cases relief comes only through a reviving of the original intolerable anxiety or the original mental breakdown.

The breakdown, this author argues, was originally caused by "an environmental factor that could not at the time be gathered into the area of the infant's omnipotence." Babies cannot identify external factors, and experience "a threat of annihilation."

If the treatment is successful, patients will be able to enact the environmental failure, and will

> experience it within the area of personal omnipotence, and so with a diminished narcissistic wound. Thus it is that as analysts we repeatedly become involved in the role of failure, and it is not easy for us to accept this role unless we see its positive value. We get made into parents who fail, and only so do we succeed as therapists. This is just one more example of the multiple paradox of the parent-infant relationship.
>
> (Winnicott, 1989 [1961], p. 75)

Mitchell (1997), in turn, expounds on the reasons that have historically led us to overlook interaction in psychoanalytic practice and on the changes that have enabled its acknowledgment. For this author, traditional theory of technique, with its emphasis on the neutral analyst, objective and remote, seems designed to belie, through an injunction, the complexity of the analyst's participation. The illusion underlying this attitude consists in thinking that the latter has no consequences for the patient or the treatment. "Rather than dealing with these issues head-on," claims Mitchell, "traditional psychoanalytic theorizing, by declaring the analytic situation a one-person field, rendered them invisible" (Mitchell, 1997, p. 11). These clinical situations, like many similar ones recorded in our own collection of anecdotes, validate N. Bleichmar and others' (2001) conclusion that psychoanalytic treatments are not concerned with curing illnesses but with favouring mental growth, which implies changing the personality structure.

Notes

1 This chapter is a modified version of the articles published in *Intercambios/ Intercambis* (November 2002) and in *Aperturas*, 13. It is also a reformulation of my contribution to the book *Winnicott hoy, su presencia en la clínica actual* [Winnicott Today, His Presence in Current Clinical Practice], edited by Liberman and Abello (Madrid: Psimática, 2008).
2 I will not discuss Freudian and post-Freudian conceptions of the setting, which are clearly explained by Etchegoyen (1999).
3 Bleichmar (1997) has advanced a *modular-transformational* model of psychic functioning that is based on the coexistence of different motivational systems such as narcissism, attachment, and sensuality/sexuality. Based on these

considerations, he argues that the psyche has "an articulated modular structure (...) [with] multiple motivational systems or modules that, in their interaction, set psychic activity in motion, check it, or give it one or another direction" (Bleichmar, 1997, p. 20). From this perspective, we no longer view unconscious functioning as homogeneous. Rather, there are different modules or systems that are generated by primary or secondary inscription, or that lack inscription, which are responsible for different modes of operation.

Zukerfeld and Zonis Zukerfeld (1999), in turn, suggest the inclusion of what they call "tertiary processes," which are very useful in present-day clinical practice. In their own words,

> it is not possible to think of psychic functioning only in terms of primary or secondary processes. We should specify that the saturated primary process corresponds to impulses and disorganized thought, and the saturated secondary process, to intellectualization and empty words (...) we reformulate the notion of tertiary process as the coming into contact with what was split or is impossible to narrate, a process that constitutes a true creation.
>
> (Zukerfeld and Zonis Zukerfeld, 1999, no pagination)

4 Bettelheim (1960, p. 36) claims that psychoanalytic therapy is essentially "a very special environment with its unique consequences," an environment that replaces the person's natural surroundings. According to this author, examining patients' reactions within this specialized environment will necessarily generate attitudes and revelations that will favour the therapy.

5 Green (1986) states that the analyst

> will respond to the empty space with an intense effort of thought in order to try to think that which the patient cannot think, and which would find expression in an effort to achieve imaginal representation on the analyst's part, so that he will not be overtaken by this psychic death.
>
> (Green, 1986, p. 42)

6 Zirlinger (2002) provides an excellent summary of the analyst's function according to Winnicott:

> ...analysts' contributions have diversified. They are not just aimed to unveil the unconscious by way of interpretation. They fulfil numerous functions, such as: accepting the transference; supporting the situation and the paradox; adapting to dependence needs and containing regression; tolerating lack of integration, senselessness, and lack of communication; presenting the object and reality; containing interpretations and emotions; enabling a state of play; mirroring; surviving; offering interpretations; retrieving reparatory gestures; accepting being used and forgotten.

And he adds:

> Some of these functions may be implicit in the rule of abstinence and suspended attention (...), but I think that his [Winnicott's] work with children and severely ill patients, and his discoveries about life and human nature, has allowed him to underscore them in this way.
>
> (Zirlinger, 2002, no pagination)

9 Relational and intersubjective psychoanalysis[1]

The intersubjective approach

Addressing the topic of intersubjectivity inevitably leads us to rethink psychic motivations, that is, our hypotheses about the construction of subjectivity. For this reason, I will start with some definitions regarding motivations and their vicissitudes. Intersubjective ideas appear in the epistemological scene of complexity in the aftermath of the structuralist boom of the mid-twentieth century. Epistemological thought ceases to focus on simplifiable objects. Moreover, it is no longer possible to make predictions based on specific or determined cause-effect phenomena or to universalize concepts, which was so reassuring to the first scientists.

Based on Heisenberg's (1930) uncertainty principle, the observer is an inseparable part of the object of study. Later will come Prigogine's work on chaos and dissipative structures (Prigogine and Stengers, 1984); theories that contemplate chance, uncertainty, and indeterminacy; and the notion of heterogeneity and the crisis of the idea of order. The first models are built that tackle phenomena from the viewpoint of complexity. To build these models, scientists must draw from a variety of disciplines. The myth of the isolated subject, of the isolated mind, is broken. In Morin's (1992) words,

> we must, then, ask ourselves if there are different complexities, and if these complexities can be connected to create a complex of complexities. We must, finally, see if there is a mode of thinking, or a method, equal to taking up the challenge of complexity. It is not a question of resuming the ambition of simple thought and controlling and dominating reality. Rather, we must train in a way of thinking that can connect, enter into a dialogue, negotiate with the real.
>
> (Morin, 2009, p. 22)

If we go back to the first psychoanalytic writings, we find a categorical Freud who, in *The Interpretation of Dreams*, unhesitatingly asserts that "nothing but a wish can set our mental apparatus at work" (Freud, 1900, p. 567). He is talking about an infantile, sexual, and perpetual desire. Two decades later, in an attempt to unite the psychoanalytic movement, Freud (1923) defines the "corner-stones" of psychoanalytic theory, which I quoted above:

> The assumption that there are unconscious processes, the recognition of the theory of resistance and repression, the appreciation of the importance of sexuality and of the Oedipus complex – these constitute the principal subject-matter of psychoanalysis and the formulations of its theory. No one who cannot accept them all should count himself a psychoanalyst.
>
> (Freud, 1923a, p. 247)

In "On Transience" (1916a), that literary gem written 15 years after the book on dreams and simultaneously with the metapsychology, he shows a somewhat more flexible facet in relation to his early radical determinism. Referring to World War I, which was raging at the time, he ends the article as follows: "We shall build up again all that war has destroyed, and perhaps on firmer ground and more lasting than before" (Freud, 1916a, p. 307). In this passage Freud encourages hope, an attitude that allows us to intuit that the apparatus he conceived may be more open to novelty, to the new, which contrasts with the well-known repetition of (inexhaustible) infantile sexual desires.

It is worth recalling here my suggestion regarding "Inhibitions, Symptoms and Anxiety" (1926d). In this essay, after emphasizing the relevance of fantasy in his metapsychology, Freud addresses the external world, the environment. He states that the human baby "is sent into the world in a less finished state." As a result, "the dangers of the external world have a greater importance for it, so that the value of the object which can alone protect it against them (…) is enormously enhanced" (pp. 154–155). These potential dangers, therefore, render the object highly significant. The authors who see the maternal figure as critical to development are bearing in mind these dangers, which logically and chronologically precede the threat of castration.

Elsewhere, Freud (1930) enumerates the three sources of psychic suffering and situates them at the same level. These sources are one's own body, the external world, and the others – one's fellow beings. In this text, unlike in others by this author, drive and object are equally seen as the cause (the source) of the dangers that beset humans. Motivation is not circumscribed to the drives. These very different quotes show a Freud who, on the one hand, tries to adapt his conception of the human psyche to the deterministic positivism of the turn of the nineteenth century, following Helmholtz. His discoveries, thus, may be considered scientific because they can be measured and reproduced. Yet on the other hand, and perhaps desperately, Freud tries to account for non-measurable, complex phenomena for which no explanation can be found.

As an example, we may quote the case history of the Wolf-Man. Here, Freud tries to introduce us into the development of an infantile neurosis, its consequences in adult life, and its treatment. The complexities of the patient are not limited to his diagnosis (we can no longer consider neurosis the right diagnosis in this case; we are dealing with one of the borderline categories). They also involve the treatment and the analyst's position in it. (It is worth recalling here that Freud had to raise money so that the patient could continue with his therapy. The psychoanalytic theory of the time could not account for this decision. Today we could see it as a response to the deficit observed in the patient's psychic structure.)

Clinical practice shows new paths for theory to take, but a dilemma emerges when the available theories only allow us to see the cross-section of the clinical material that confirms them. Going beyond this cross-section, immersing ourselves in contradiction, and trying to understand the new field lying before us is what makes our discipline grow. This is the right time to remember how theories of subjectivity are developed. They are the product of:

1   the creator's empirical basis;
2   the society and the times in which he or she lives; and
3   his or her own personality, biography, and history.

Since theory is a powerful tool, moreover, its development also depends on the power/knowledge dynamics within and without scientific institutions. Therefore, faced with a theoretical conceptualization, we analyse its content by taking into account the clinical starting point, the time when it was created, and the creator. This combination of factors will result in a product that will always be perishable. It will lack an expiration date, but times evolve, as do creators. We can see this evolution in relation to Freud's theories of anxiety, narcissism, and the drives.

Freud chooses the Oedipus myth and its consequences to depict the structuring of the psyche in order to illustrate what he sees as the cornerstone of psychoanalysis. We know that myths have manifold versions and change over time, for they are always viewed/constructed with materials chosen from the observer's point of view. Freud's particular version focuses on the crossroads, on that scene where the inter-generational struggle (Oedipus vs. Laius) is staged, as well as on its clinical by-products – hostility, rivalry, and jealousy. For the many reasons discussed earlier (biographical, historical, geographical, and related to scientific development), Freud takes this part of the myth and not the part of which this one is a consequence – Oedipus's helplessness in the face of his parents' abandonment.

What part of the myth could be considered most representative of today's urban humans? Haven't schizoid and borderline personalities (gestated in failed encounters and nurtured by absence) displaced last century's hysterics? We have characterized our contemporary urban empirical base as populated by patients who are "empty, alexithymic, dissociated," with whom it is impossible to operate based on a hysteric (tripartite) view of object relations. Yet we should conduct joint studies with sociologists and other researchers of social events, especially concerning the prevalence of ephemeralness and instability in emotional relationships. There is a vast literature that addresses these issues. Some of these works discuss the nature of postmodernity, among them, Vattimo (1992), Gergen (1991), López Gil (1992), Lyotard (1992), Casullo et al. (1999), and Bauman (2003).

Green (1995) considers that Freud's work

> is the reflection of a practice that was defined in a historically determined social field (...) his discoveries are necessarily tied, in part, to the sociohistorical determinations of his time. This does not mean that these determinations suffice to downplay the significance of his work. Rather, it means that this work is traversed by determination from beginning to end. If our practice changes, psychoanalysis changes, which means that when sociohistorical conditions change, analysands and analysts change as well, and hence their relations and dynamic, topographical, and economic modes of exchange necessarily alter.
>
> (Green, 1995, pp. 223–224)

One of the schools that emerged between the third and fourth decades of the last century built on a line of thinking that goes from the Hungarian school to Winnicott, and gave rise to present-day intersubjective thinkers. Doubtless, prioritizing the environment has led me to focus on psychoanalytic thought models that view not only the vicissitudes of the drives but also the objects provided by the environment as indispensable for human development. In these models, furthermore, the absence, failure, or inadequate functioning of these objects has a great influence on the aetiology of illnesses.

As a consequence, the Oedipal conflict ceases to be the only cause of pathology. Even if we supplement them with narcissistic vicissitudes, we still need to consider other factors that participate in the structuring and activation of the psyche, factors that interrelate in a complex web. As I pointed out earlier, it is impossible to find an explanatory tool, a metapsychology that is comprehensive enough to encompass all these factors. Bleichmar, hence, attempted to integrate into our field the knowledge produced by the neurosciences and cognitive psychology, and adopted a modular approach.[2]

One of the most prolific authors in intersubjective theory is Lichtenberg (1996). Lachmann and Fosshage outline ten key issues that summarize Lichtenberg's approach to intersubjective clinical practice (Freire and Moreno, 1999). Analysts should promote a friendly, conscious, and reliable relationship between patient and analyst, and apply empathy to reassure or stimulate the patient. They should also describe the patient's experience in detail. According to Lichtenberg, transferences are new creations stemming from the intersubjective field and, largely, from unconscious communications; patients perceive interferences on the part of the analyst of which he or she is unaware. Model scenes serve as an example. These scenes may be brought in by patient or analyst and may have a range of sources – memories, dreams, imagination, films, or novels. The goal is to reconstruct not repressed memory but current purposes. The interest of the scene lies not in its reconstruction but in its conceptual potential. We must attach proper significance to aversive motivations and refrain from interpreting them as a defence or an avoidance strategy. When we explore an affect or any emotional content, we should go as far as the patient is able to experience it and not any farther.

Lichtenberg (1989) categorically stresses that motivations only arise from lived experience, and that vitality depends on the ways in which emotionally charged exchanges unfold between children and their caregivers. Bacal (1998) also rejects the idea that the therapeutic aspect of psychoanalytic treatment is insight resulting from interpretation. The therapeutic effect of this treatment hinges on a relational experience with a therapist who is prepared to respond both to patients' unique suffering and to their efforts to achieve their particular life goals in different ways that are therapeutically specific.

Another of the most renowned intersubjectivists (even though he defined himself as a relationalist) is Mitchell, who died young. He argues that all meaning is produced within relationships, and hence nothing is innate, as the drive model suggests. This author points out that the most elemental bodily events, such as hunger, bowel movements, and orgasms, are experienced through the symbolic texture of the relational matrix and are interpreted in that context. Broadly, therefore, the very establishment of the relational matrix is innate, and perhaps it would be better to define human development as "a continuous unfolding of an intrinsically determined social nature" (Stern, 1985, p. 234).

Mitchell justifies his argument by pointing out that relational-model theories share a vision that is very different from Freud's, and have "changed the nature of psychoanalytic inquiry." This vision portrays humans

> not as a conglomeration of physically based urges, but as being shaped by and inevitably embedded within a matrix of relationships with other people, struggling both to maintain our ties to others and to differentiate ourselves from them. In this vision the basic unit of study is (…) an interactional field within which the individual arises and struggles to make contact and to articulate himself. *Desire* is experienced always *in the context of relatedness*, and it is that context which defines its meaning. Mind is composed of relational configurations.
>
> (Mitchell, 1988, pp. 3–4; author's emphasis)

People, therefore, can only be understood within this tapestry of past and present relationships. Analysts' task requires that they participate in this tapestry and, at the same time, that they observe, reveal, and transform it and its representations in patients' minds. The figure, claims Mitchell, "is always the tapestry and the threads of the tapestry (via identifications and introjections)" (ibid., 4).

For this author, there is no isolated "self" in a psychological sense outside the relational matrix. In the relational model, he adds,

> the repetitive patterns within human experience are not derived, as in the drive model, from pursuing gratification of inherent pressures and pleasures (nor, as in Freud's post-1920 understanding, from the automatic workings of the death instinct), but from a pervasive tendency to preserve the continuity, connections, familiarity of one's personal, interactional world. There is a powerful need to preserve an abiding sense of oneself as associated with, positioned in terms of, related to, a matrix of other people, in terms of actual transactions as well as internal presences.
>
> (1988: 33)

Mitchell believes that understanding the past allows us to find clues to decipher how and why the present is configured the way it is. These initial experiences are not "structural remainders." They are important because they constitute the first representation of relationships that will be repeated time and time again under different guises in later developmental phases. The goal of analysis is to change patients' relational modes.

Stolorow and Atwood, who are the most conspicuous exponents of the intersubjective school, assert that

> the specific intersubjective contexts in which conflict takes form are those in which central affect states of the child cannot be integrated because they fail to evoke the requisite attuned responsiveness from the caregiving surround. Such unintegrated affect states become the source of life-long inner conflict, because they are experienced as threats both to the person's established psychological organization and to the maintenance of vitally needed ties. Thus affect-dissociating defensive operations are called into play, which reappear in the analytic situation in the form of resistance (...) It is in the defensive walling off of central affect states, rooted in early derailments of affect integration, that the origins of what has traditionally been called the dynamic unconscious can be found.
>
> (Stolorow et al., 1987, pp. 91–92)

"From this perspective," these authors claim, "the dynamic unconscious is seen to consist not of repressed instinctual drive derivatives, but of affect states that have been defensively walled off because they evoked massive malattunement from the early surround" (Stolorow and Atwood, 1992, p. 184). What leads to the development of children's sense of reality is not frustration and disappointment but empathic validation provided by their surroundings. Such validation depends on the existence of emotional attunement, which gives rise to a range of positive and negative experiences that are emotionally charged. Reality, then, is the product of an interface of emotionally attuned subjectivities.

The absence of empathic validation at different stages of development may lead to the appearance of disorders, for children must adapt the organization of their experiences to the experiences of their caregiver so as to protect a bond that is essential to their well-being. As they are able to communicate symbolically and become aware of others as subjects, excessive adaptation may cause their subjective world to be constituted largely by a foreign reality that has been imposed from the outside.

This lengthy introduction is necessary to tackle the current notion of intersubjectivity. To do so, we must revisit basic theoretical and clinical concepts. In intersubjective theory, the unconscious is no longer viewed as a drive reservoir, a concept that is close to biology. Instead, it is approached from the perspective of alterity. Rather than biology/culture, the equation is now unit/alterity, a shift that involves a relational reformulation of the nature of the unconscious. The intersubjective approach does not focus on endogenous instinctive forces but on remainders of alterity (of complex interactions with other people through presence and care, affects developed in a relationship, and so on) as unconscious formations.

This approach was already germinating in some of Freud's writings, especially in "Inhibitions, Symptoms and Anxiety," and was developed in different ways by the Hungarian school (Ferenczi, Balint), by members of the British school (Fairbairn, Bowlby, Winnicott, Bollas, and M. Kahn), by North American thinkers (Kohut, Gedo, Goldberg, Modell, Ogden, and the above-quoted Stolorow, Atwood, and Mitchell, and by Orange in its philosophical foundations), as well as by independent theoreticians with different origins and trainings (McDougall, Killingmo, Berenstein, Puget, and Bleichmar). We should probably also add Liberman, Pichon-Rivière, and Bleger, who made major contributions to the intersubjective perspective.

These new, provocative ways of thinking about the psyche are the product of social phenomena that participate in the current construction of subjectivity; contemporary life, perplexity, indeterminacy, and uncertainty have given rise to new paradigms that, in turn, have shaped diverse approaches to and ways of conceptualizing psychoanalysis. Intersubjectivity means envisioning subjects who are open to their history, their present, and their future, who live in the paradox inherent in the repetition-vs.-newness equation. Subjectivity is constituted in a process of becoming. It is not only repetition, re-edition; it is edition as well. It is not just re-presentation but also presentation. It is not mere release and search for equilibrium; it is also a search for objects and complexity. Intersubjectivists consider that subjects are open to their culture and marked by events.

The intersubjectivist approach views psychoanalytic treatment as the co-creation by patient and analyst of a safe environment that, based on a continuous meeting, will facilitate an intense, deep joint exploration of unconscious aspects and make possible the edition of unlived or novel situations. Co-creation depends on the analyst-patient relationship and its context. It is not universal, and transcends the traditional debate on *via di porre* vs. *via di levare* by advancing a third option, the *via di creare*, which includes both members of the analytic couple (Oelsner, personal communication).

To end this chapter, I will say, along with Riera (2001), that if we can think of parricidal Oedipus as a child who was abandoned by its parents and of Narcissus as a teenager who needs a gaze that will integrate his or her self and rescue him or her from disintegration; if we admit that the analyst is not a blank slate or someone who provides good milk rejected by envy, evil, or the deflection of the death instinct of the guilty patient; if we think of the differences between Oedipal desires and early needs; and finally, if we think of patients as eager to be understood by their analyst and not just as repressing infantile desires, our practice may be called intersubjective analysis.

Notes

1 In our discipline, the term intersubjectivity was coined by Stolorow, Atwood, and Ross in 1978. Today, more than three decades later, this perspective has greatly developed. For a glimpse into the breadth and quality of the field, see the various volumes of *Relational Psychoanalysis*, published by The Analytic Press.

2 Going back to Bleichmar's (1997) modular-transformational approach, we can say that it is a technique with specific therapeutic interventions that is active, targeted, and flexible in its manifold modes of intervention. Along with the key role of making conscious the unconscious, it emphasizes the importance of procedural memory, cognitive restructuring, changes in the patient's actions, and exposure to new experiences. Psychotherapy should be tailored to each case and guided by the following questions: What type of interventions? For what subtype of psychopathological syndrome? For what personality structure? For what life moment? For what treatment conditions (long-duration or brief psychotherapy, psychotherapy in private practice or in institutions, family therapy, and so on)? It is a psychotherapy that is not limited to trying to modify symptoms. In addition, it attempts to change personality traits that cause suffering – automatisms in interpersonal relations that are present since childhood, are beyond patients' control, and disturb their everyday life. It is based on a psychopathology that strives to overcome reductionism and single-cause explanations, for these explanations overlook the manifold motivational systems that promote fantasy and acts. This psychopathology describes subtypes of depressive disorders, narcissistic disorders, anorexia, borderline disorders, substance abuse, conditions that activate aggressiveness, masochism, gender identity disorders, sexuality disorders, and so on.

10 Psychiatry after Winnicott[1]

Psychiatry is at present essentially a descriptive and classificatory science whose orientation is still towards the somatic rather than the psychological and which is without the possibility of giving explanations of the phenomena which it observes. Psycho-analysis does not, however, stand in opposition to it, as the most unanimous behaviour of the psychiatrists might lead one to believe. On the contrary, as a *depth-psychology*, a psychology of those processes in mental life which are withdrawn from consciousness, it is called upon to provide psychiatry with an indispensable groundwork and to free it from its present limitations. We can foresee that the future will give birth to a scientific psychiatry, to which psychoanalysis has served as an introduction.

(Freud, 1923A, p. 251).

I have been invited to refer to psycho-analytic treatment, and to balance this a colleague has been invited to refer to individual psychotherapy. I expect we both start off with the same problem: how to distinguish between the two? Personally I am not able to make this distinction. For me the question is: has the therapist had an analytic training or not?

Winnicott (1958, p. 115)

The context, the eras, the professionals

Winnicott's legacy includes a series of concepts and tools that enable us to examine our work, our clinical practice in more depth. As it is to be expected with any scientific development, paradigmatic ideas transcend the life and work of the person who formulates them. Concepts develop, expand, and are looked at from the perspective of other practices that are influenced by the sociocultural context, and hence seem different over time. They are now closer to the historical archive than to clinical work.

When we mention Winnicott's contributions, we are probably being unfair to many other psychoanalytic authors whose ideas make up the core conceptions of what I would like to call "the Self School" (because of the broad common ground between Winnicott and Kohut's perspectives and those of their followers, even if Kohutians claim this name for themselves).

In earlier chapters I stated, perhaps repeatedly, that every original author draws from the ideas of his or her time and of his or her precursors. This "plagiarism" is inevitable. How could we quote Winnicott without recognizing in his work Buber or Bergson's philosophical ideas or the clinical contributions of Ferenczi, Fairbairn, or Klein? Or quote Kohut without finding in his work Hartmann, Mahler, or Erikson's concepts?

Of course, we cannot consider every contribution because authors emerge from a dialectic spiral that includes their past, their personal history, their family, their teachers, their patients, their practices, in sum, their milieu, with its legal framework and also its myths (as they are told and interpreted at that time). If they have creative ideas to offer, they will be acknowledged by their peers for their original contributions. Such recognition goes beyond these authors' written work to include the oral history woven around them (what they never wrote but we assume they would have thought) and the imaginary surrounding their lives and work. These elements, moreover, will also shape the ways in which these authors are viewed outside their community.

As Winnicott taught us, the preconditions for the true self are the spontaneous gesture and the personal idea, and this self will only materialize if it finds a significant fellow being who can mirror that created gesture and fully bring it to life. It is precisely the other's mirroring, the mother's face, which blends with the initial gesture of the developing subject, that renders the study of context indispensable. Such context is incessantly being created by a radical and necessary intersubjectivity, and constitutes a basic paradigm to understand Winnicott's contributions. From this perspective, it is worth reiterating, developing subjectivities need the other to acquire their own unique traits. This other is not a mere reflection; he or she is a real person, function, and context. Like Winnicott, Kohut attributes a key role to this dialectic.

I will not characterize our current times, and the changes we have witnessed to daily life, as postmodern (although this characterization has been used, perhaps in excess). Being slightly arbitrary, I believe we can point to the end of World War II as the beginning of our age – after Auschwitz, or after Freud's death. I have already addressed the role of history in the subjectivation process. It is also at this time that psychiatry starts benefiting from psychoanalysis. Today we can find a large population of colleagues worldwide who combine these two disciplines in both their private practice and their teaching. Psychoanalysis intertwines with psychiatry in a continuum that has wide (and sometimes unstable) borders.

I myself am an example of this phenomenon, for my own development occurs in a permanent interaction between these two disciplines; their boundaries are not easily discernible in my practice. Yet we can be sure that psychoanalysis offers psychiatric practice a tool that is as valuable as it is irreplaceable, for it enables psychiatrists to access patients' psychic world beyond the surface and to understand their subjective architecture. In this way, based on the notion of complemental series, psychiatrists can assess subjects' interaction with their environment, their family, and their everyday activities. All these components are inherent in patients – none of this is foreign to them.

I have noticed that even if we adhere to diverse frames of reference, psychoanalytically trained psychiatrists cannot avoid looking at our clinical work from a psychoanalytic perspective. This viewpoint is integrated into the diagnostic process and involves a professional attitude that is expressed in the psychiatrist's position regarding the patient.[2] At the same time, today we will rarely find a physician or psychologist who has trained only as a psychoanalyst. Mental health practitioners learn early on that, as Maslow said so well, "it is tempting, if the only tool you have is a hammer, to treat everything as if it were a nail" (Maslow, 1966, pp. 15–16). Consequently, before they become mature psychoanalysts, they travel different paths or, at least, look at mental pathology from different viewpoints. It is not surprising that those who train as analysts have previously been taught cognitive or systemic therapies or have prescribed drugs, and they often continue to pursue these other modes of training in parallel to their psychoanalytic career.

It is worth going back to Winnicott's query in the quote above: "For me the question is: has the therapist had an analytic training or not?" It is not an easy question to answer, especially these days, when analytic training is hard to define.

An excerpt of my personal history (or how I started using Winnicott)

I discovered Winnicott's work after finishing my basic training in psychiatry, and he has been part of my frame of reference ever since. While my clinical work has benefited from the experience acquired over the years, I do not think it is very different from the work I did as a resident at the Lanús Hospital. Of course, today I have more elements to ponder and conceptualize my practice. Being slightly ironic about myself, I could say I have reached a place that is near my point of departure. I simply try to theorize while preserving the pragmatic aspect of clinical acts, dismissing pure speculation, looking at patients as inseparable from their surroundings, and viewing symptom relief as necessary in order to make progress in the therapeutic relationship.

During the psychotherapy or psychoanalytic session, I try to keep in mind how important it is for patients to be heard and to be remembered by what they say and do. This therapeutic attitude affects patients' self-esteem regulation; it allows them to preserve a narcissism that is suitable for survival without needing to distort their self or resort to complex defensive ego structures. Therefore, besides seeing manifest content as a guide to latent content, I try to value it per se. It is not always a defence or a screen, since patients stage their situation through it. Therefore, we need to understand it. I try to distance myself from interpretive options such us, "What you actually wanted to say..." or "Behind what you're saying...," which downplay patients' ability to communicate and demand an unnecessary splitting for patients to acquire the knowledge with which they will expand the field of their consciousness.

As I grew professionally, I understood that the feeling of hatred, sometimes expressed as aggression, is not a basic affect, a motivation. Rather, it is a consequence of fear, neglect, and abuse (we already knew that they were not just fantasies!). In some cases, it may also stem from an identification with fearful or aggressive early objects whose behaviour toward the patient was similar to the behaviour recreated in the session. At the Lanús Hospital I learned excellent practices, many of which have not been conceptualized. As I was able to understand later on, these practices were based on a frame of reference that closely resembles Winnicott's ideas on mental health, especially in what concerns the significance of the mother figure and the family and his notions of health and illness, which I described earlier. Winnicott explains these notions in the books he wrote for the general public: *The Child and the Outside World* (1957) *The Family and Individual Development* (1965c), *Talking to Parents* (1993), and *Babies and Their Mothers* (1987).

It is worth recounting some personal experiences that will help to explain my current approach, which builds on my hospital years, my early practice, and the ideas of the authors who became my favourites over time. Not long after I finished the excellent residency at the Psychiatry Ward of the Lanús Hospital, this hospital was taken over by a military physician appointed by the military dictatorship. An assistant to the military officer in charge confessed to me that their goal was to "put an end to the homosexual, Jewish, Marxist, and psychoanalyst Lanús hospital." (This strategy was not new. It had a precedent in the decades-old insidious opposition to Goldenberg, the director of the ward, and his innovative conceptions. To reveal the truth behind this statement, however, we should open a bracket before "homosexual" and close it after "psychoanalyst.")

Why this attack on Goldenberg's ward? During his training as a psychiatrist, Goldenberg was greatly influenced by psychoanalysts with an excellent psychiatric training, such as Enrique Pichon-Rivière and Celes Cárcamo. Then he unhesitatingly brought in to teach courses prestigious members of the recently established Argentine Psychoanalytic Association, like Grinberg, Liberman, Zac, Itzigsohn, and Caparrós. As early as 1950, during the first international psychiatric conference, his curiosity, always so keen, drove him to meet Melanie Klein and Anna Freud, as well as Henri Ey and López Ibor (Diamant, 2005). The dictatorship viewed the new concepts arising from this "melting pot of ideas" as subversive.

Teaching psychiatry at the Lanús Hospital was always "glued" to clinical practice. It was (and still is for those who trained there) a way of working with mental health patients. We described and theorized, but speculation was secondary to therapeutic practice. In this sense, and maybe this is an exaggeration, technique was the variable. We could not systematize it, but this drawback became an advantage, because we could adjust it in response to lessons learned in our work. We were quite clear about what we should not do, though not so much about what we should do. We discussed our approach with our peers, with the chief resident, or with more experienced colleagues. In addition, we conveyed as best we could the ineffable situations we experienced with our patients to prestigious analysts who came to the hospital as supervisors.

We had to deal with severe pathologies stemming from lack of stimuli, abuse, and neglect, all of which led to the development of a deficient structure. It was rare to find a typical neurotic conflict. Medical histories were populated with disorders stemming from environmental problems that had affected patients since very early on – both absence of care and disturbing presences. Neglect and abandonment were particularly common. We could verify the lack of an elemental and continuously present support network that, had it existed, would have allowed patients to develop their psyche without disruption. As a treatment, we provided psychotherapy with or without medication and group or family therapy. Back then, we coined the notion of institutional transference to describe the bond that tied the patient to the service and its conceptions rather than to one of the practitioners.

In our debates, we did not conceive of an evidence-based science. What is "evident" tends to prevail as a bias that blocks the ability to develop intersubjective thinking over the course of a treatment.[3] In this sense, a prognosis based on the patient's psychopathology, or even on his or her therapeutic past, will not aid to the evolution of the treatment. If we protect ourselves from such knowledge, our prospects will likely be better. Zukerfeld and Zonis Zukerfeld (2004) carried out a valuable study that shows that analysts who do not take into account patients' history operate differently. They free themselves from deterministic prejudices and improve their prospects, and hence also their therapeutic outcome.

Without making small differences into narcissistic bastions, my conclusion is that I do not see great dissimilarities between a good psychoanalytically trained psychiatrist and a good psychoanalyst.

Winnicott's contribution, especially in what concerns severely ill patients

If it is difficult to systematize Winnicott's work, it is also hard to examine his contributions in a methodical way. In my experience and in the experience of colleagues who know his work well, it is clear that psychiatry has been greatly enriched by his and his followers' ideas. If they were a work of art, these ideas would bear the signature of several authors spanning a few decades. Winnicott's contributions to the understanding and treatment of psychosis and other severe pathologies, which I already discussed elsewhere

(Nemirovsky, 1999), have greatly enhanced our grasp of the psychological aspects of these pathologies (whose chemical features have been clarified in recent years, thanks to input from research into the chemistry of the brain). Not many analysts work regularly with this type of patient, and Winnicott's writings offer great insight as to aetiology in the case of patients who have suffered significant interruption to the continuity of their existence in early childhood (patients with severe neuroses, borderline personalities, and psychoses).

When reflecting on the severity of the pathologies they are tackling, psychiatrists could profit from concepts developed by the different psychoanalytic schools. If they based their diagnosis on Freud's theory of repression, they would consider that a severely ill patient is someone who, after repeated interventions, cannot distinguish memory from transference. If their reference point were Bleger (1967), they would focus on the agglutinated aspects of the personality and their glischro-caric anchorage. If they were familiar with Masud Khan's work, they would view patients' history in terms of the breaches in the protection of the self described by this author in connection with the notion of cumulative trauma.

If they used McDougall's (1980) ideas as a starting point, they would consider that severely ill patients are those who have suffered severe trauma. Or, they would focus on the patient as non-represented if they were drawing from Botella and Botella (1997). They might also resort to contributions made by Klein, Fromm-Reichman, Bion, or Resnik. And if they based their diagnosis on Winnicott (1971), they would think of severely ill patients as those who failed to develop a transitional space. Over the course of the treatment, the progress of the therapy could be assessed through the development of a space for play between the protagonists.

Psychiatrists' attitude, in terms of their devotion to the case, is also an important diagnostic indicator. Therapists' concern differs depending on the bond they establish with the patient. They will find that there are patients who need to be kept constantly in mind (and often demand attention very loudly). In these cases, psychiatrists could resort to Winnicott's notion of primary maternal preoccupation, which would help them understand the role of first objects in human development. It is through practitioners' concern that many patients' lacks emerge in the therapeutic field, and such concern often provides the only opportunity for patients to receive what the environment never gave them (Nemirovsky, 1999).

If they have been well trained, psychiatrists will be aware, based on their experience and knowledge, that at first a severely ill patient will need them to prioritize the inflection and the tone of their voice, and the timeliness rather than the content of their interventions. They will also know that the hardest patients to treat are particularly alert to para-interpretive aspects of verbal communication. In this regard, Winnicott's ideas provide many elements to conceptualize the various aspects of communication in relation to metaphorical and actual holding.

In psychiatric practice, the notion of setting we have discussed so far – a setting that supports, protects, and gives hope – is very useful and of great clinical significance. We often need to establish a supporting "network" with family, friends, and co-workers or with therapeutic companions. This network constitutes a frame (analogous to the mother-baby relationship) that facilitates the establishment of communication with the therapist. The notions of *holding* and *handling* will hence be very useful to understand the role played by it. In this sense, if they have developed a positive bond with the patient, internists will be another important figure in the configuration of the holding. If we deem it necessary, we will communicate with them, give them the place they deserve in the patient's affects, and make them into allies.

The same is true when a psychologist leads the treatment. Communication with him or her and with other members of the network should be smooth and ongoing so as to avoid gaps in the therapeutic structure concerning medication or other issues managed by the psychiatrist. If psychiatrists plan on using psychotropic drugs, it is worth recalling Ferrali's (1977) advice on the matter. This author reminds us that medicating is part of a comprehensive therapeutic process, and takes place within a relationship based on words. Medications may be viewed as signs that make up a "communicative package." This package comprises a chemical signal that acts on the brain's biological structure; a symbol, "which links beliefs, expectations, and attitudes of giver and receiver" (a dynamic that includes the transference relationship); and a social symbol, which is tied to the social imaginary.

Ferrali thus distinguishes among three different concepts:

-the drug as a pure chemical signal;
    -the placebo, a symbolic principle of the binary and social channel that is pharmacologically empty; and
    - the medicine, which meets the three requirements of chemical signal, symbol of the binary channel, and social symbol, and becomes what it is through the entirety of its signifying nature.

(Ferrali, 1977, p. 32)

This carefully thought-out approach to medication sheds light on the manifold roles of the pharmacological tool and combines different perspectives, including psychoanalysis. Gabbard's (2005) comments on drug prescription are also appropriate:

One patient experienced the prescription of an antidepressant as an empathic failure on the part of the psychiatrist. When the patient's non-compliance was explored with him, he told his doctor, 'I was looking for someone to validate my feelings. Instead, you tried to medicate them away.'

(Gabbard, 2005, p. 144)

The empathic bond will guide us to decide, along with the patient, whether or not to use drugs.

Let us turn now to other elements in Winnicott's work that are useful to psychiatrists. When a priest asked him for guidance as to when he should refer someone to psychological treatment during confession, Winnicott told him that he should recommend treatment when his parishioner bored him. Here Winnicott is suggesting a very useful bond-related diagnostic tool tied to the countertransference, and recommends looking at the main aspect of the notion of health, that is, the vitality of the self. More specifically, he is pointing to the perception of such vitality in a flesh-and-blood subject. The opposite of vitality is "chronic boredom," which expresses numbness, non-life.

Winnicott sets forth the continuity of existence as a health paradigm in several essays. Such continuity is based on humans' innate tendency toward growth, while mental illness constitutes the arrest of development. In the case of severely ill patients, therefore, we must remove the obstacles to development so that individuals may grow, thanks to their inherited potential. In this sense, Winnicott's simple taxonomy is very useful for psychiatrists. He argues that there are different categories of patients depending on the technical equipment the analyst must use in their treatment, as I mentioned earlier.

Yet it is worth highlighting that when treating pre-depressive, severely ill, or complex subjects, we must be very patient and try to empathize with their affective states so that we can reconstruct their fragmented history based on the transference bond. Moreover, when patients demand an additional hour, we need to take their attitude into account, and we will have to perform many tasks besides being there without interpreting. I already mentioned that Winnicott suggests prioritizing interpretation in "deep" pathologies and in relation to the deep aspects of patients in whom early deficiencies prevail. The deepest aspects will appear only if we facilitate resolution through the development of what failed to evolve during their early childhood. In this regard, it is worth referring to Winnicott's classic article "Fear of Breakdown" (Winnicott, 1974).

Other essential contributions by this author are associated with the concept of self. It is very important for psychiatrists to distinguish true (original and personal, stemming from spontaneous gestures and personal ideas) from false (arising from subjects' identification with the other). During the diagnostic phase, to achieve the right therapeutic approach, practitioners must differentiate between what the patient *is* from what belongs to others and "fills the emptiness." In other words, they must separate what belongs to the patient from what corresponds to a defence. (It is in this context that Winnicott emphasizes the word *false* to allude to what does not genuinely belong to the patient and can be pathological when impermeable, that is, when it isolates instead of protecting the self and enables submission or the flight to health.)

We should not forget the notion of psychotherapy as a space for shared play that Winnicott formulates in *Playing and Reality* (1971). The configuration of a space that allows for virtuality and creation is certainly one of the goals of any useful therapeutic modality. There are still many contributions by Winnicott to discuss; I have only enumerated the ones that I see as critical. At the same time, it would not make sense, except from a pedagogical perspective, to write an endless list that would hinder psychiatrists' individual elaboration of this author's work. I would like to end by stressing a concept that was dear to him and that is essential to determine our position regarding the patient. Winnicott repeatedly points out that people cannot show themselves just as they are, in their absolute intimacy – they cannot wear their heart on their sleeve (Winnicott, 1960b, p. 143).

Practitioners should keep in mind these specific features of the therapeutic meeting when they ponder their participation in a treatment. They must constantly face this paradox, which, as such, constitutes a dilemma requiring an ethical answer – approaching the patient in order to make contact while respecting his or her intimacy. Furthermore, these concepts are germane not only to the question of communication between psychiatrist and patient but also to the use of medication or other therapeutic tools (hospitalization, therapeutic accompaniment). Whatever tool we employ, we must be alert to patients' specificities and refrain from forcing them to change. Only thus will they achieve a healthier life. In the case of many severely ill patients, as we often must accept, the only thing we can do is support them and try to remove the obstacles that are hampering their development.

Notes

1 This chapter is a reformulation of my contribution to the book *Winnicott hoy, su presencia en la clínica actual* (Winnicott Today, His Presence in Current Clinical Practice), edited by A. Liberman and A. Abello, Madrid: Psimática, 2009.

2 Those practitioners who do not consider the cure the goal of every analysis and, more specifically, those who do not value symptomatic relief will probably disagree with this point of view. We could say that it is an ethical position according to the Chilean analyst Varela's (1992) definition of ethics. This author points out that ethics is neither a behaviour, nor an acquisition of the ego, nor a technique, nor the knowledge of rules and procedures. It is not based on judgement or reason but on an immediate confrontation with the facts. It depends on the development of an "ethical skill" as a disposition "to act not according to reason but to wisdom," and cannot be learned. It consists of ordinary, spontaneous actions based on the contemporary perception that there is no stable or transcendental ego.

3 In their study on drug testing in psychiatry, S. Levin and M. Nemirovsky (2004) state that nowadays, knowledge on psychopharmacological therapeutics is mostly obtained by conducting controlled clinical trials. These trials are critical to evidence-based medicine (EBM), which has become the prevalent mode of clinical thinking. "Most medical schools and healthcare providers," the authors argue, "have adopted EBM with increasing enthusiasm." Providers view EBM

as a potential ally in cost reduction processes. It was believed that EBM would help eliminate ineffective and costly procedures and, by combining practice and evidence, costs would be reduced. Costs, however, kept rising, and EBM (...) started to be used as a powerful marketing argument (powerful in it is 'scientifically valid'). We believe that the knowledge of the terms of this debate is particularly relevant in these times, when the hegemony of evidence discourse in the medical field has transformed criticism into a marginal practice. While there is no doubt that modern psychopharmacology has improved the prognosis of many mental ailments, we need to challenge the status of 'indisputable discourse' with which it tends to be presented.

(Levin and Nemirovsky, 2004, p. 6)

References

Ades, D. (1982). *Dalí and Surrealism*. New York: Harper & Row.

Aguilar, J. R. (2000). *Déficit y conflicto* [Deficit and Conflict], unpublished.

Anzieu, D. (1959). *El autoanálisis de Freud y el descubrimiento del psicoanálisis*. Mexico: Siglo XXI, 1987 [*Freud's Self-Analysis*. Translated by P. Graham. London: Hogarth Press and the Institute of Psycho-analysis, 1986].

Anzieu, D. (1974). Le moi-peau. *Nouvelle Revue de Psychanalyse*, **9**: 195–208 [*The Skin-Ego: A Psychoanalytic Approach to the Self*. Translated by C. Turner. London: Karnac, 1989].

Aragonés, R. J. (1999). *El narcisismo como matriz de la teoría* [Narcissism as a Matrix for Theory]. Buenos Aires: Nueva Visión.

Aslan, C. M. (1988). El fundamento común en psicoanálisis: fines y procesos clínicos. *Rev. de Psicoanálisis*, **45**(4): 735–742 [Common ground in psychoanalysis: Aims and clinical process. As I see it. *Int. J. Psychoanal.*, **34**(3): 573–583].

Atwood, G. E. and Stolorow, R. D. (1984). *Structures of Subjectivity: Explorations in Psychoanalytic Phenomenology*. Hillsdale, NJ: The Analytic Press.

Atwood, G. E. and Stolorow, R. D. (1993). *Faces in a Cloud: Intersubjectivity in Personality Theory*. Northvale, NJ: Jason Aronson.

Avenburg, R. (1984). *El desarrollo psíquico temprano tal como se refleja en el proceso psicoanalítico* [Early psychic development as reflected in the psychoanalytic process]. *Psicoanálisis*, **6**(2–3): 233–242.

Bacal, H. A. (Ed). (1998). *Optimal Responsiveness: How Therapists Heal Their Patients*. Northvale, NJ: Jason Aronson Inc.

Bacal, H. A. and Thomson, P. G. (1996). Las necesidades de selfobject del psicoanalista y el efecto de su frustración en el curso del tratamiento: una nueva visión de la contratransferencia. *Intercambios: papeles de psicoanálisis*, **1**: 67–78 [The psychoanalyst's selfobject needs and the effect of their frustration on the treatment: A new view of countertransference. In: Goldberg, A. (Ed.), *Basic Ideas Reconsidered: Progress in Self Psychology* (pp. 17–35). Hillsdale, NJ: The Analytic Press, 1996.

Balint, M. (1957). *The Doctor, His Patient, and the Illness*. New York: International Universities Press.

Balint, M. (1968). *The Basic Fault: Therapeutic Aspects of Regression*. London: Tavistock Publications.

Baranger, W. (1969). El narcisismo en la obra de Freud. In: Sandler, J. (Ed.), *Estudios sobre "Introducción al narcisismo" de Sigmund Freud*. Madrid: Julián Yebenes, 1991 [Narcissism in Freud. In: Sandler, J., Spector Person, E. and Fonagy, P. (Eds.), *Freud's "On Narcissism: An Introduction"* (pp. 108–130). New Haven, CT: Yale University Press, 1991].

Baranger, M. and Baranger, W. (1969). *Problemas del campo psicoanalítico*. Buenos Aires: Kargieman [The analytic situation as a dynamic field. *Int. J. Psychoanal.*, **89**: 795–826, 2008].

Bauman, Z. (2003). *Amor líquido*. Buenos Aires: F.C.E., 2005 [*Liquid Love: On the Frailty of Human Bonds*. Cambridge, UK: Polity Press].

Benyakar, M. (2003). *Lo disruptivo* [Disruptiveness]. Buenos Aires: Biblos.

Bergsson, G. (2004). *La magia de la niñez* [The Magic of Childhood]. Translated by E. Bernardez. Barcelona: Tusquets.

Bettelheim, B. (1960). *El corazón bien informado. La autonomía en la sociedad de masas*. Mexico, DF: Fondo de Cultura Económica, 1973 [*The Informed Heart: Autonomy in a Mass Age*. Glencoe, IL: The Free Press].

Bettelheim, B. (1967). *La fortaleza vacía*. Barcelona: Laia, 1972 [*The Empty Fortress: Infantile Autism and the Birth of the Self*. New York: The Free Press].

Bettelheim, B. (1986). Vienne 1880–1939. Guía de la Exposición del C. George Pompidou [*Freud's Vienna and Other Essays*. New York: Knopf, 1990].

Bleger, J. (1967). *Simbiosis y ambigüedad. Estudio psicoanalítico*. Buenos Aires: Paidós [*Symbiosis and Ambiguity: A Psychoanalytic Study*. Edited by J. Churcher and L. Bleger. Translated by J. Churcher, L. Bleger, and S. Rogers. Routledge, 2012].

Blake, W. (s/d). *The Marriage of Heaven and Hell*. Boston, MA: J. W. Luce and co., 1906.

Bleichmar, H. (1997). *Avances en psicoterapia psicoanalítica* [Advances in Psychoanalytic Psychotherapy]. Buenos Aires: Paidós.

Bleichmar, H. (2000). Aplicación del enfoque "Modular-Transformacional" al diagnóstico de los trastornos narcisistas [Applying the Modular-Transformational approach to the diagnosis of narcissistic disorders]. *Aperturas*, 5. Retrieved from: http://www.aperturas.org/articulos.php?id=123&a=Aplicacion-del-enfoque-Modular-Transformacional-al-diagnostico-de-los-trastornos-narcisistas.

Bleichmar, N. and Bleichmar, C. (1989). *El psicoanálisis después de Freud. Teoría y clínica* [Psychoanalysis after Freud: Theory and Practice]. Mexico, DF: Eleia.

Bleichmar, N., Leiberman de Bleichmar, C., Matarasso, S., Salazar, J., Cacher, M. L., Cardós, G., Islas, C., Lozano, G. and Ortiz, E. (2001). *Las perspectivas del psicoanálisis* [Perspectives in Psychoanalysis]. Mexico, DF: Paidós.

Borges, J. L. (1975). *El libro de arena*. Buenos Aires: Emecé [*The Book of Sand*. Translated by Norman Thomas di Giovanni. New York: Dutton, 1977].

Borgogno, F. (2005). Llegar a ser: la importancia de la respuesta afectiva del analista a los sueños de una paciente esquizoide deprivada emocionalmente. *Aperturas*, 20. Retrieved from: http://www.aperturas.org/articulos.php?id=335&a=Llegar-a-ser-la-importancia-de-la-respuesta-afectiva-del-analista-a-los-suenos-de-una-paciente-esquizoide-deprivada-emocionalmente [On the patient's becoming an individual: The importance of the analyst's personal response to a deprived schizoid patient. In: *The Girl Who Committed Hara-Kiri and Other Clinical and Historical Essays*. Translated by Alice Spence (pp. 3–29). London: Karnac, 2013].

Botella, C. and Botella, S. (1997). *Más allá de la representación* [Beyond Representation]. Valencia: Promolibro.

Bouvet, M. (1968). *La relation d'object* [Object Relations]. Paris: Payot.

Bowlby, J. (1940). The influence of early environment in the development of neurosis and neurotic character. *Int. J. Psychoanal.*, **21**: 1–25.

Bowlby, J. (1951). *Maternal Care and Mental Health: A Report Prepared on Behalf of the World Health Organization as a Contribution to the United Nations Programme for the Welfare of Homeless Children.* Geneva: World Health Organization.

Bowlby, J. (1969). *Attachment and Loss, Vol. I. Attachment.* London: The Hogarth Press.

Bowlby, J. (1979). Psychoanalysis as art and science. *Int. Rev. Psychoanal.*, 6(1): 3–14.

Broucek, F. J. (1991). *Shame and the Self.* New York: Guilford.

Carr, E. H. (1961). *¿Qué es la historia?* Buenos Aires: Sudamericana, 1984 [*What Is History?* New York: Vintage].

Casullo, N., Forster, R. and Kaufman, A. (1999). *Itinerarios de la modernidad* [Itineraries of Modernity]. Buenos Aires: Eudeba.

Croce, B. (1996). *Historia de Europa en el siglo XIX.* Barcelona: Ariel [*History of Europe in the Nineteenth Century.* Translated by Henry Furst. New York: Harcourt, Brace and Co., 1933].

Davis, M. and Wallbridge, D. (1981). *Límite y espacio.* Buenos Aires: Amorrortu, 1988 [*Boundary and Space: An Introduction to the Work of D. W. Winnicott.* London: Brunner-Routledge].

Diamant, A. (Ed.) (2005). Mauricio Goldenberg: El maestro del Lanús [Mauricio Goldenberg, "el Lanús" Teacher]. *Avances en Salud Mental Relacional / Advances in Relational Mental Health*, 4(2): 1–6.

Dio de Bleichmar, E. (1977). Psicopatología de la infancia [Childhood psychopathology]. In: Vidal, G., Bleichmar, H. and Usandivaras, R. (Eds.), *Enciclopedia de psiquiatría* [Encyclopedia of Psychiatry]. Buenos Aires: El Ateneo.***

Dio de Bleichmar, E. (2002). Sexualidad y género: nuevas perspectivas en el psicoanálisis contemporáneo [Sexuality and gender: New perspectives in contemporary psychoanalysis]. *Aperturas*, 11. Retrieved from: http://www.aperturas.org/articulos.php?id=202.

Dupetit, S. (1988). Convergencias de teorías psicoanalíticas: apuntes para una posible discusión [Convergences in psychoanalytic theory: Notes for a potential discussion]. In: Parres, R. (Ed.), *Psicoanálisis, Convergencia de teorías Psicoanálisis y poder Desarrollo temprano. Memorias del XVI Congreso Latinoamericano de Psicoanálisis y del XI Pre-Congreso Didáctico. Tomo I* [Proceedings of the 16th Latin American Psychoanalytic Conference: Psychoanalysis, Convergence of theories – Psychoanalysis and Power – Early Development. Volume I]. Mexico, DF: Federación Psicoanalítica de América Latina (FEPAL).

Eco, U. (1984). *The Name of the Rose.* Translated by William Weaver. New York: Harcourt.

Emde, R. (1988). Development terminable and interminable. *Int. J. Psychoanal.*, 69: 23–42.

Erikson, E. H. (1950). Growth and crises of the "healthy personality." In: Senn, M. J. (Ed.), *Symposium on the Healthy Personality* (pp. 91–146). New York: J. Macy, Junior Foundation.

Erikson, E. H. (1982). *El ciclo vital completado.* Buenos Aires: Paidós, 1985 [Erikson, E. and Erikson, J. M. *The Life Cycle Completed, Extended Version.* New York: W. W. Norton, 1997].

Etchegoyen, R. H. (1986). *Los fundamentos de la técnica psicoanalítica. 2da edición.* Buenos Aires: Amorrortu, 2002 [*The Fundamentals of Psychoanalytic Technique, Revised Edition.* Translated by Patricia Pitchon. London: Karnac, 1999].

Etchegoyen, R. H. (1990). El psicoanálisis de la última década. La clínica y la teoría. Ficha de la Asociación Psicoanalítica de Buenos Aires [Psychoanalysis in the last decade: Clinical and theoretical aspects. *Psychoanal. Enq.*, **11**(1): 88–106].

Ey, H. (1978). *En defensa de la psiquiatría* [In Defense of Psychiatry]. Translated by A. Pagés Larraya. Buenos Aires: Huemul, 1979.

Fairbairn, W. R. (1941). A revised psychopathology of the psychosis and psychoneurosis. *Int. J. Psychoanal.*, **4**: 751–781.

Fairbairn, W. R. (1952). *Estudio psicoanalítico de la personalidad.* Buenos Aires: Hormé, 1962 [*Psychoanalytic Studies of the Personality.* London and New York: Routledge, 2001].

Fairbairn, W. R. (1954). Observaciones sobre la naturaleza de los estados histéricos. In: Saurí, J. J. (Ed.), *Las histerias.* Buenos Aires: Nueva Visión, 1985 [Observation on the nature of hysterical states. *Br. J. Med. Psychol.*, **27**(3): 105–125].

Fenichel, O. (1945). *Teoría psicoanalítica de las neurosis.* Buenos Aires: Paidós, 1966 [*The Psychoanalytic Theory of Neurosis.* New York: W.W. Norton].

Ferenczi, S. (1927). *Teoría y técnica del psicoanálisis.* Buenos Aires: Paidós, 1967 [*Further Contributions to the Theory and Technique of Psychoanalysis.* Edited by J. Rickman and translated by J. Suttie and others. New York: Boni and Liveright].

Ferenczi, S. (1928). Elasticidad de la técnica psicoanalítica. In: *Psicoanálisis Vol IV* (pp. 59–72). Madrid: Espasa Calpe, 1984 [The elasticity of psycho-analytic technique. In M. Balint (Ed.) and E. Mosbacher and others (trans.), *Final Contributions to the Problems and Methods of Psycho-Analysis* (pp. 87–101). London: Hogarth Press, 1955].

Ferenczi, S. (1929). El niño mal recibido y su impulso de muerte. *O.C. Vol IV.* Madrid: Espasa-Calpe, 1984 [The unwelcome child and his death instinct. In: *Final Contributions to the Problems and Methods of Psycho-Analysis* (pp. 102–107). London: Hogarth Press, 1955].

Ferenczi, S. (1933). Confusión de lenguajes entre los adultos y el niño. *O.C. Vol. IV.* pp. 139–149. Madrid: Espasa-Calpe, 1984 [Confusion of tongues between the adult and the child. *Int. J. Psychoanal.*, **30**: 225–230, 1949].

Ferenczi, S. (1988). *Diario clínico.* Buenos Aires: Conjetural [*The Clinical Diary of Sándor Ferenczi.* Edited by J. Dupont and translated by M. Balint and N. Z. Jackson. Cambridge, MA: Harvard University Press].

Ferrali, J. C. (1977). Fobia social. Estudio en el contexto de los trastornos de ansiedad en general y de las fobias en particular [Social phobia: Study in the context of anxiety disorders in general and phobias in particular]. *Desarrollos en Psiquiatría Argentina*, **2**(3): 22–27.

Ferrater Mora, J. (1984). *Diccionario de filosofía* [Dictionary of Philosophy]. Madrid: Alianza.

Fiorini, H. (1999). *Nuevas líneas en psicoterapias psicoanalíticas: teoría, técnica y clínica* [New Lines in Psychoanalytic Psychotherapies: Theory, Technique, and Clinical Practice]. Madrid: Psimática.

Freire, B. and Moreno, E. (1999). Reseña de [Review of] *The Clinical Exchange: Techniques Derived from Self and Motivational Systems* (1996). *Aperturas*, 1. Retrieved from: http://www.aperturas.org/articulos.php?id=57&a=The-clinical-exchange-Techniques-derived-from-self-and-motivational-systems-1996.

Freud, A. (1965). *Normalidad y patología en la niñez.* Buenos Aires: Paidós, 1971 [*Normality and Pathology in Childhood: Assessment of Development.* New York: International Universities Press, 1965].

Freud, S. (1900). *La interpretación de los sueños*, Vol. IV. Buenos Aires: Amorrortu, 1977 [The Interpretation of dreams (first part). *S.E.*, **4**: ix–627].

Freud, S. (1912). *La dinámica de la transferencia*, Vol. XII. Buenos Aires: Amorrortu, 1977 [The dynamics of transference. *S.E.*, **12**: 97–108].

Freud, S. (1915). Pulsiones y destinos de pulsión, Vol. XIV. Buenos Aires: Amorrortu, 1977 [Instincts and their vicissitudes. *S.E.*, **14**: 111–140].

Freud, S. (1916a). La transitoriedad, Vol. XIV. Buenos Aires: Amorrortu, 1977 [On transience. *S.E.*, **14**: 303–310].

Freud, S. (1916b). *Conferencias de Introducción al Psicoanálisis, Parte III*, Conf. n. 26, La teoría de la libido y el narcisismo, Vol. XV. Buenos Aires: Amorrortu, 1977 [Lecture XXVI: The libido theory and narcissism. In: *Introductory Lectures on Psycho-Analysis. S.E.*, **16**: 412–430].

Freud, S. (1918). *De la historia de una neurosis infantil*, Vol. XVII. Buenos Aires: Amorrortu, 1977 [From the History of an Infantile Neurosis. *S.E.*, **17**: 3–124].

Freud, S. (1920). Más allá del principio del placer, Vol. XVIII. Buenos Aires: Amorrortu, 1977 [Beyond the Pleasure Principle. *S.E.*, **18**: 3–66].

Freud, S. (1923). Dos artículos de enciclopedia: Psicoanálisis y Teoría de la libido, Vol. XVIII. Buenos Aires: Amorrortu, 1977 [Two encyclopaedia articles. *S.E.*, **18**: 234–262].

Freud, S. (1926). *Inhibición, síntoma y angustia*, Vol. XX. Buenos Aires: Amorrortu, 1977 [Inhibitions, symptoms and anxiety. *S.E.*, **20**: 77–178].

Freud, S. (1930). *El malestar en la cultura*, Vol. XXI. Buenos Aires: Amorrortu, 1977 [Civilization and its discontents. *S.E.*, **21**: 59–148].

Freud, S. (1933). *Nuevas conferencias de introducción al psicoanálisis*, Vol. XXII. Buenos Aires: Amorrortu, 1985 [New introductory lectures on psychoanalysis. *S.E.*, **22**: 3–184].

Freud, S. (1950). *Proyecto de psicología* (1895), Vol. I. Buenos Aires: Amorrortu, 1977 [Project for a scientific psychology. *S.E.*, **1**: 281–391].

Gay, P. (1988). *Freud, una vida de nuestro tiempo*. Barcelona: Paidós, 1989 [*Freud, A Life of Our Time*. New York: W.W. Norton, 1988].

Gabbard, G. (2005). *Psiquiatría psicodinámica en la práctica clínica*. Buenos Aires: Panamericana [Psychodynamic Psychiatry in Clinical Practice, Fourth Edition. Arlington, VA: American Psychiatric Association Publishing].

Galli, V. (1982). Una perspectiva de investigación psicoanalítica en psicosis [An approach to psychoanalytic research into psychosis]. *Actas del XIV Congreso Psicoanalítico de América Latina* [Proceedings of the 14th Latin American Psychoanalytic Conference]. Buenos Aires: FEPAL.

Gedo, J. and Goldberg, A. (1973). *Modelos de la mente*. Buenos Aires: Amorrortu, 1980 [*Models of the Mind: A Psychoanalytic Theory*. Chicago: The University of Chicago Press].

Geets, C. (1993). *Donald Winnicott*. Buenos Aires: Almagesto.

Gergen, K. J. (1992). *El Yo saturado*. Buenos Aires: Paidós [*The Saturated Self: Dilemmas of Identity in Contemporary Life*. New York: Basic Books, 1991].

Ginzburg, C. (1989). Morelli, Freud y Sherlock Holmes: indicios y método científico. In: *El signo de los tres* (pp. 55–99). Barcelona: Lumen [Clues: Roots of an evidential paradigm. In: *Clues, Myths, and the Historical Method*. Translated by John and Anne Tedeschi (96–125). Baltimore: Johns Hopkins University Press, 1992].

Gioia, T. (1984). El miedo ¿emoción básica? [Fear: Basic emotion?] *Psicoanálisis*, **2–3**: 555–582.

Gioia, T. (1996). *Psicoanálisis y etología* [Psychoanalysis and Ethology]. Buenos Aires: Typos.

Giovacchini, P. (1972). *Tactics and Techniques in Psychoanalytic Therapy, Vols. 1 and 2.* New York: Jason Aronson.

Green, A. (1975). *De locuras privadas.* Buenos Aires: Amorrortu, 1990 [*On Private Madness.* London: Hogarth, 1986; reprinted Karnac 1997].

Green, A. (1986). *Narcisismo de vida, narcisismo de muerte.* Buenos Aires: Amorrortu [*Life Narcissism, Death Narcissism.* Translated by Andrew Weller. London: Free Association Books, 2001].

Green, A. (1995). *La metapsicología revisitada* [Metapsychology Revisited]. Buenos Aires: EUdeBA, 1996.

Grinker, R., Werble, B., and Drye, R. (1968). *The Borderline Syndrome.* New York: Basic Books.

Guntrip, H. (1967). The concept of psychodynamic science. *Int. J. Psychoanal.,* **48**(1): 32–43.

Guntrip, H. (1971). *El self en la teoría y la terapia psicoanalíticas.* Buenos Aires: Amorrortu, 1973 [*Psychoanalytic Theory, Therapy and the Self.* New York: Basic Books].

Guntrip, H. (1975). My experience of analysis with Fairbairn and Winnicott: (How complete a result does psychoanalytic therapy achieve?). *Int. J. Psychoanal.,* **77**: 739–754.

Hartmann, H. (1939). *Ego Psychology and the Problem of Adaptation.* New York: International Universities Press.

Hartmann, H. (1970). *Ensayos sobre la psicología del yo.* Mexico, DF: Fondo de Cultura Económica [*Essays on Ego Psychology: Selected Problems in Psychoanalytic Theory.* New York: International Universities Press, 1965].

Heisenberg, W. (1930). *The Physical Principles of the Quantum Theory.* Translated by C. Eckart and F. C. Hoyt. Chicago: University of Chicago Press.

Hoffmann, J. M. (1984). El desarrollo temprano del Self [Early development of the self]. *Psicoanálisis,* **6**(2/3): 261–294.

Hoffmann, J. M. (1999). Preservar la espontaneidad vs. acatamiento: un aspecto interaccional del desarrollo temprano [Preserving spontaneity vs. compliance: An interactional aspect of early development]. In: Lancelle, G. (Ed.), *El self en la teoría y en la práctica* [The Self in Theory and Practice] (pp. 251–290). Buenos Aires: Paidós.

Home, H. J. (1966). El concepto de la mente. *Rev. de Psicoanálisis,* **26**(1) [The concept of mind. *Int. J. Psychoanal.,* **47**: 42–49].

Jiménez Avello, J. (1998). *Para leer a Ferenczi* [Reading Ferenczi]. Madrid: Biblioteca Nueva.

Joffe, W. G. and Sandler, J. (1967). Some conceptual problems involved in the consideration of disorders of narcissism. *J. Child Psychother.,* **2**(1): 56–66.

Jordán, J. F. (2001). Experiencia, trauma y recuerdo. A propósito de un texto de Winnicott [Experience, trauma and memories: Concerning a text by Winnicott]. *Gradiva,* **3**(2): 157–164.

Jordán, J. F. (2010). Mutuo reconocimiento y el uso del objeto. Del filósofo en su silla a Donald. Winnicott [Mutual recognition and the use of the object: From the philosopher on his chair to Donald Winnicott]. *Rev. Chilena de Psicoanálisis,* **27**(2): 113–116.

Juri, L. and Ferrari, L. (2000). ¿Rivalidad edípica o cooperación intergeneracional? Del Edipo de Freud al Ulises de Kohut [Oedipal rivalry or intergenerational cooperation? From Freud's Oedipus to Kohut's Ulysses]. *Aperturas*, 5. Retrieved from: http://www.aperturas.org/articulos.php?id=0000118.

Kaplan, H. and Sadock, B. (1994). *Sinopsis de psiquiatría*. Buenos Aires: Panamericana, 1996 [*Kaplan and Sadock's Synopsis of Psychiatry: Behavioral Sciences Clinical Psychiatry*. Baltimore: Williams and Wilkins, 1988].

Kernberg, O. (1975). *Desórdenes fronterizos y narcisismo patológico*. Mexico: Paidós, 1993 [*Borderline Conditions and Pathological Narcissism*. New York: Jason Aronson].

Khan, M. and Masud, R. (1958). Introduction. In: Winnicott, D. W. (Ed.), *From Paediatrics through Psychoanalysis* (pp. xi–l). New York: Basic Books.

Khan, M. and Masud, R. (1963). El concepto de trauma acumulativo. In: *La intimidad del sí-mismo* (pp. 47–66). Madrid: Saltes, 1980 [The concept of cumulative trauma. In: *The Privacy of the Self* (pp. 42–58). London: The Hogarth Press, 1974].

Killingmo, B. (1989). Conflict and deficit: Implications for technique. *Int. J. Psychoanal.*, **70**: 65–79.

Koestler, A. (1981). *Jano*. Madrid: Debate [*Janus: A Summing Up*. New York: Random House, 1978].

Kohut, H. (1959). Introspection, empathy, and psychoanalysis. *JAPA*, **7**: 459–483.

Kohut, H. (1966). Forms and transformation of narcissism. *JAPA*, **14**: 243–272.

Kohut, H. (1971). *Análisis del self*. Buenos Aires: Amorrortu Editores, 1977 [*The Analysis of the Self*. New York: International Universities Press].

Kohut, H. (1977). *The Restoration of the Self*. New York: International Universities Press.

Kohut, H. (1979). The two analyses of Mr. Z. *Int. J. Psychoanal.*, **60**: 3–27.

Kohut, H. (1982). Introspection, empathy and the semi-circle of mental health. *Int. J. Psychoanal.*, **63**: 395–413.

Kohut, H. (1984). *¿Cómo cura el análisis?* Buenos Aires: Paidós, 1986 [*How Does Analysis Cure?* Edited by A. Goldberg. Chicago: The University of Chicago Press].

Kozer, J. (2005). Lo hermoso fluye sin espacio. Entrevisto por Jorge Luis Arcos [Beauty flows without space: Interview with Jorge Luis Arcos]. *Encuentro de la cultura cubana*, **37–38**: 24–34.

Lancelle, G. (1984). Desarrollo psíquico temprano y psicología psicoanalítica del self. Reseña de los puntos de vista de Heinz Kohut [Early psychic development and psychoanalytic psychology of the self: Overview of Heinz Kohut's viewpoints]. *Psicoanálisis*, 6(2–3): 451–461.

Lancelle, G. (Ed.) (1999). *El self en la teoría y en la práctica* [The Self in Theory and Practice]. Buenos Aires: Paidós.

Lancelle, G., Lerner, H., Nemirovsky, C., and Ortiz Fragola, A. (1990). Las identificaciones propias e impropias en el psicoanalizar [Proper and improper identifications in psychoanalytic practice]. *Psicoanálisis*, 12(1): 83–103.

Laplanche, J. (1987). *Nuevos fundamentos para el psicoanálisis. La seducción originaria*. Buenos Aires: Amorrortu [*New Foundations for Psychoanalysis*. Translated by David Macey. Oxford: Basil Blackwell, 1989].

Laplanche, J. and Pontalis, J-B. (1967). *Diccionario de Psicoanálisis*. Barcelona: Labor, 1968 [*The Language of Psycho-Analysis*. Translated by D. Nicholson-Smith. London: The Hogarth Press, 1973].

Laurent, É. (2004). Hijos del trauma [Children of trauma]. In: Belaga, G. (Ed.). *La urgencia generalizada: la práctica en el hospital* [Generalized Emergency: Practicing in the Hospital] (pp. 23–29). Buenos Aires: Grama.

Leclaire, S. (1977). La transferencia/Transference. Lecture at the Argentine Psychoanalytic Association, Buenos Aires.

Lerner, H. (2001). *El psicoanálisis es terapéutico* [Psychoanalysis is therapeutic]. Retrieved from: www.apdeba.org.

Lerner, H. and Nemirovsky, C. (1989a). La empatía en el psicoanalizar [Empathy in psychoanalytic work]. *Psicoanálisis*, 11(1): 129–143.

Lerner, H. and Nemirovsky, C. (1989b). Personalidad borderline: déficit estructural y problemas clínicos [Borderline personality: Structural deficit and clinical problems]. Presented at APdeBA's Eleventh Symposium, Buenos Aires, November.

Lerner, H. and Nemirovsky, C. (1990). La estructuración del self como cambio psíquico [The structuring of the self as psychic change]. Presented at APdeBa's Twelfth Symposium, Buenos Aires, November.

Lerner, H. and Nemirovsky, C. (1992). La clínica del déficit. Relación con su origen traumático [Deficit in clinical practice: Relationship with its traumatic origin]. Presented at APdeBA's Fourteenth Symposium Buenos Aires, November.

Levín de Said, A. (2000). Regresión a la dependencia [Regression to dependence]. Presented at Encuentro Winnicott, Rio de Janeiro, October.

Levín, S. and Nemirovsky, M. (2004). Controversias en torno del ensayo clínico controlado de psicofármacos [Controversies around the controlled clinical trial of psychotropic drugs]. Unpublished.

Levinton, N. (2001). Relacionalidad. Del apego a la intersubjetividad. [Book review of *Relationality: From Attachment to Intersubjetivity*]. *Aperturas*, No. 4. Retrieved from: http://www.aperturas.org/articulos.php?id=185&a=Relacionalidad-Del-apego-a-la-intersubjetividad.

Lebovici, S. (1994). Empathie et "enactment" dans le travail de contre-transfert [Empathy and enactment in countertransference work]. *Revue Française de Psychanalyse*, **58**: 1551–1561.

Lichtenberg, J. D. (1989). *Psychoanalysis and Motivation*. Hillsdale, NJ: The Analytic Press.

Lichtenberg, J. D., Lachmann, F. and Fosshage, J. L. (1996). *The Clinical Exchange: Techniques Derived from Self and Motivational Systems*. Hillsdale, NJ: The Analytic Press.

Lipovetsky, G. (1986). *La era del vacío* [The Era of Emptiness]. Translated by Joan Vinyoli and Michèle Pendanx. Barcelona: Anagrama.

López Gil, M. (1992). *Filosofía, modernidad, posmodernidad* [Philosophy, Modernity, Postmodernity]. Buenos Aires: Biblos.

Loewald, H. (1978). Primary process, secondary process, and language. In: *Papers on Psychoanalysis* (pp. 178–206). New Haven: Yale University Press, 1980.

Lyotard, J. F. (1994). *La posmodernidad (explicada a los niños)*. Buenos Aires: Gedisa [*The Postmodern Explained to Children: Correspondence 1982–1985*. Translated by J. Pefanis and M. Thomas. Sidney: Power Publications, 1992].

Mahler, M. (1968). *Simbiosis humana: las vicisitudes de la individuación*. Buenos Aires: Paidós [*On Human Symbiosis and the Vicissitudes of Individuation*. New York: International Universities Press].

Mahler, M., Pine, F., and Bergman, A. (1975). *El nacimiento psicológico del infante humano*. Buenos Aires: Marymar, 1977 [*The Psychological Birth of the Human Infant: Symbiosis and Individuation*. New York: Basic Books].

Marrone, M. (2001). *La teoría del apego* [Attachment Theory]. Madrid: Psimática.

Maslow, A. (1966). *The Psychology of Science*. New York: Harper & Row.

McDougall, J. (1980). *Plea for a Measure of Abnormality*. New York: International Universities Press.

McDougall, J. (1987). *Teatros de la mente*. Madrid: Tecnipublicaciones [*Theaters of the Mind: Illusion and Truth on the Psychoanalytic Stage*. New York: Basic Books, 1985].

Meltzer, D. (1975). Adhesive identification. *Contem. Psycho-Anal.*, **11**(3): 289–310.

Mitchell, S. A. (1988). *Conceptos relacionales en psicoanálisis, una integración*. Mexico, DF: Siglo XXI, 1993 [*Relational Concepts in Psychoanalysis: An Integration*. Cambridge, MA: Harvard University Press].

Mitchell, S. A. (1991). Contemporary perspectives on self: Toward an integration. *Psychoanal. Dialog.*, **1**(2): 121–147.

Mitchell, S. A. (1997). *Influence and Autonomy in Psychoanalysis*. New York: Taylor & Francis.

Mitchell, S. A. (2000). *Relationality: From Attachment to Intersubjectivity*. Hillsdale, NJ: The Analytic Press.

Modell, A. (1984). *Psychoanalysis in a New Context*. New York: International Universities Press.

Moguillansky, R. (1992). Conferencia de homenaje al Dr. M. Goldenberg [Tribute to Dr. M. Goldenberg]. Lecture, ApdeBA, Buenos Aires, August.

Morin, E. (2009). *Introducción al pensamiento complejo* [Introduction to Complex Thought]. Translated by Marcelo Pakman. Barcelona: Gedisa.

Nemirovsky, C. (1993). ¿Otros analistas, otros pacientes? Reflexiones acerca del psicoanálisis actual [Other analysts, other patients? Reflections on present-day psychoanalysis]. Presented at the 28th IPA Congress, Amsterdam, July.

Nemirovsky, C. (1997). Algunas reflexiones (polémicas) acerca del pensamiento de D.W. Winnicott sobre las psicosis [Some (polemical) reflections about the ideas of D. W. Winnicott on psychoses]. Presented at the VI Latin American Meeting on D. W. Winnicott's Ideas, Buenos Aires, November.

Nemirovsky, C. (1999). Edición-Reedición. Reflexiones a partir de los aportes de Winnicott a la comprensión y tratamiento de las psicosis y otras patologías graves [Edition-reedition: Reflections based on Winnicott's contributions to the understanding and treatment of psychoses and other severe pathologies]. *Aperturas*, 3. Retrieved from: http://www.aperturas.org/articulos.php?id=0000089.

Nemirovsky, C. (2001). Las perspectivas de Winnicott y de Kohut en el psicoanálisis [Winnicott and Kohut's perspectives in Psychoanalysis]. *Aperturas*, 7. Retrieved from: http://www.aperturas.org/articulos.php?id=149&a=Las-perspectivas-de-Winnicott-y-de-Kohut-en-el-psicoanalisis. Published also in *Psicoanálisis*, **24**(3): 501–520, 2002.

Nemirovsky, C. (2003). Encuadre, salud e interpretación. Reflexiones alrededor de conceptos de D. W. Winnicott [The setting, health and interpretation: Reflections about D.W. Winnicott's concepts]. *Aperturas*, 13. Retrieved from: http://www.aperturas.org/articulos.php?id=233&a=Encuadre-salud-e-interpretacion-Reflexiones-alrededor-de-conceptos-de-DWWinnicott.

Nietzche, F. (1972). *La gaya ciencia, libro tercero*. [*The Gay Science*. Translated by Thomas Common. Minneola, NY: Dover Publications, 2006].

Oelsner, R. (1988). Notas sobre el trauma precoz y la transferencia: el viaje desde ninguna parte [Notes on early trauma and the transference: The journey from nowhere]. *Revista de psicoanálisis*, **46**(5): 784–797.

Orange, D. M., Atwood, G. E., and Stolorow, R. D. (1997). *Working Intersubjectively*. Hillsdale, NJ: The Analytic Press.

Ortiz Fragola, A. (1999). La angustia y el happening [Anxiety and happenings]. In: Lancelle, G. (Ed.), *El self en la teoría y en la práctica* (pp. 235–249). Buenos Aires: Paidós.

Painceira, A. (1997). *Clínica psicoanalítica. A partir de la obra de Winnicott* [Psychoanalytic Practice: Starting from Winnicott's Work]. Buenos Aires: Lumen.

Painceira, A. (2002). Hacia una nueva teorización del psicoanálisis a partir de la "intuición fundamental" de Winnicott [Toward a new theorization of psychoanalysis based on Winnicott's "core intuition"]. *Psicoanálisis*, **24**(3): 521–542.

Paz, C. A. (1969). Reflexiones técnicas sobre el proceso analítico en los psicóticos [Technical reflections on the analytic process with psychotic patients]. *Revista de Psicoanálisis*, **26**(3): 571–630.

Paz, M. A. (2005). Verguenza, narcisismo y culpa en psicoanálisis [Shame, narcissism, and guilt in psychoanalysis]. *Aperturas*, 21. Retrieved from: http://www.aperturas.org/articulos.php?id=0000356.

Pelento, M. L. (1992). Apuntes sobre la obra de Winnicott [Notes on Winnicott's work]. Presented at the first Winnicott Meeting, Buenos Aires, November.

Pine, F. (1990). *Drive, Ego, Object, and Self: A Synthesis for Clinical Work*. New York: Basic Books.

Pontalis, J-B. (1971). Prólogo [Prologue]. In: Winnicott, D. W. (Ed.), *Realidad y juego* [Playing and Reality] (pp. i–viii). Barcelona: Gedisa, 1982.

Prigogine, I. and Stengers, I. (1984). *Order Out of Chaos: Man's New Dialogue with Nature*. New York: Bantam Books.

Puget, J. (1991). Entrevistando a psicoanalistas. Reportaje del Dr. M. Spivacow [Interviewing psychoanalysts: Interview with Dr. M. Spivacow]. *Psicoanálisis*, **13**(2): 391–403.

Renik, O. (1996). Los riesgos de la neutralidad. *Aperturas*, 10, March 2002 [The perils of neutrality. *Psychoanal. Q.*, **65**(3): 495–517].

Ricoeur, P. (1977). The question of proofs in Freud's psychoanalytic writings. *JAPA*, **25**(4): 853–871.

Ridruejo, D. (1971). La crítica creadora de Luis Rosales [The creative criticism of Luis Rosales]. *Cuadernos Hispanoamericanos*, **257–258**: 396–409.

Riera, R. (2001). Transformaciones en mi práctica psicoanalítica [Transformations in my psychoanalytic practice]. *Aperturas*, 8. Retrieved from: http://www.aperturas.org/articulos.php?id=0000158&a=Transformaciones-en-mi-practica.

Robbins, M (1983). Toward a new mind model for the primitive personalities. *Int. J. Psychoanal.*, **64**: 127–148.

Rodman, R. (Ed.) (1987). *The Spontaneous Gesture: Selected Letters of D. W. Winnicott*. Cambridge, MA: Harvard University Press.

Rodulfo, M. (1992). *El niño del dibujo. Estudio psicoanalítico del grafismo y sus funciones en la construcción temprana del cuerpo* [The Child of the Drawing: Psychoanalytic Study of Graphics and its Role in the Early Construction of the Body]. Buenos Aires: Paidós.

Rosenfeld, H. (1965). *Psychotic States*. New York: International Universities Press.

Rosenfeld, H. (1979). Psicosis de transferencia en pacientes borderline. APdeBA Summary of *Borderline Advances*, edited by J. Leboit and Capponi (1978). [Transference psychosis in the borderline patient. In: Leboit, J. and Capponi, A. (Eds.), *Advances in Psychotherapy of the Borderline Patient* (pp. 485–510). New York: Jason Aronson].

Roussillon, R. (1991). *Paradojas y situaciones fronterizas del psicoanálisis* [Paradoxes and Borderline Situations in Psychoanalysis]. Translated by I. Agoff. Buenos Aires: Amorrortu, 1995.

Sabina, J. (1990). Con la frente marchita [With withered forehead], December 20, 1990. *Mentiras piadosas* [White Lies], Sony U.S. Latin, CD B000005LDH.

Searles, H. (1966). *Escritos sobre esquizofrenia.* Barcelona: Gedisa [*Collected Papers on Schizophrenia and Related Subjects.* New York: International Universities Press, 1965].

Segal, F. (2005). ¿Cómo se construye la fortaleza en el ser humano? [How is strength developed in human beings?] Presented at the IV Rosario ADEP Meeting: "Vulnerabilidad y fortaleza en el campo psicoanalítico" [Vulnerability and Strength in the Psychoanalytic Field].

Shane, E. and Shane, M. (1990). Object loss and self object loss: A consideration of self psychology's contribution to understanding mourning and the failure to mourn. *Ann. Psychoanal.*, **16**: 115–131.

Schur, M. (1972). *Sigmund Freud.* Barcelona: Paidós, 1980 [*Freud: Living and Dying.* London: Hogarth Press and The Institute of Psychoanalysis].

Smalinsky, E., Ripesi, D., and Merle, E. (2009). *Winnicott para principiantes* [Winnicott for Beginners]. Buenos Aires: Era Naciente.

Stern, D. (1985). *El mundo interpersonal del infante.* Buenos Aires: Paidós, 1991 [*The Interpersonal World of the Infant: A View from Psychoanalysis and Developmental Psychology.* New York: Basic Books].

Stolorow, R. and Atwood, G. (1992). *Contexts of Being. The Intersubjetive Foundations of Psychological Life.* Hillside, NJ: The Analytic Press.

Stolorow, R., Atwood, G., and Brandchaft, B. (1987). *Psychoanalytic Treatment: An Intersubjective Approach.* Hillsdale, NJ: The Analytic Press.

Strachey, J. (1923). Introducción a *El Yo y el ello.* In: Freud, S. (Ed.), *Obras Completas* T. XIX. Buenos Aires: Amorrortu, 1976 [Introduction. In: Freud, S. (Ed.), *The Ego and the Id. S.E.*, **19**: ix–xiii].

Sullivan, H. S. (1953). *La teoría interpersonal de la psiquiatría.* Buenos Aires: Psique, 1974 [*The Interpersonal Theory of Psychiatry.* New York: W.W. Norton].

Tolpin, M. (1978). Self-objects and oedipal objects: A crucial developmental distinction. *Psychoanal. Study Child*, **33**(1): 167–186.

Valeros, J. (1997). *El jugar del analista* [The Analyst's Playing]. Mexico, DF: Fondo de Cultura Económica.

Valeros, J. (2005). Trauma en la obra de John Bowlby [Trauma in John Bowlby's work]. *Psicoanálisis*, **27**(1–2): 205–207.

Varela, F. (1992). *La habilidad ética* [The Ethical Skill]. Barcelona: Debate.

Vattimo, G. (1990). *La sociedad transparente.* Buenos Aires: Paidós [*The Transparent Society.* Translated by David Webb. London: Polity Press, 1992].

Wallerstein, R. (1983). Self psychology and "classical" psychoanalytic psychology: The nature of their relationship. *Psychoanal. Contemp. Thought*, **6**(4): 553–595.

Wallerstein, R. (1988). One psychoanalysis or many? *Int. J. Psychoanal.*, **69**: 5–21.

Watzlawick, P. (1976). ¿Es real la realidad? Barcelona: Herder, 1994 [*How Real Is Real?* New York: Random House].

Winnicott, D. W. (1945). Desarrollo emocional primitivo. In: *Escritos de pediatría y psicoanálisis.* Barcelona: Laia, 1979 [Primitive emotional development. *Int. J. Psychoanal.*, **26**(3–4): 137–143].

132   *References*

Winnicott, D. W. (1952). La psicosis y el cuidado de los niños. In: *Escritos de pediatría y psicoanálisis*. Barcelona: Laia, 1979 [Psychosis and child care. *Br. J. Med. Psychol.*, **26**: 68–74].

Winnicott, D. W. (1954). Metapsychological and clinical aspects of regression within the psycho-analytical set-up. *Int. J. Psychoanal.*, **36**: 16–26.

Winnicott, D. W. (1955–1956). Variedades clínicas de la transferencia. In: *Escritos de pediatría y psicoanálisis*. Barcelona: Laia, 1979 [Clinical varieties of transference. *Int. J. Psychoanal.*, **37**: 386–388].

Winnicott, D. W. (1956). Preocupación maternal primaria. In: *Escritos de pediatría y psicoanálisis*. Barcelona: Laia, 1979 [Primary maternal preoccupation. In: *Collected Papers: Through Paediatrics to Psychoanalysis* (pp. 300–305). London: Karnac, 1992].

Winnicott, D. W. (1957). *The Child and the Outside World*. London: Tavistock.

Winnicott, D. W. (1958). Sobre la contribución al psicoanálisis de la observación directa del niño. In: *Los procesos de maduración y el ambiente facilitador*. Buenos Aires: Paidós, 1993 [On the contribution of direct child observation to psychoanalysis. In: *The Maturational Processes and the Facilitating Environment: Studies in the Theory of Emotional Development* (pp. 109–114). New York: International Universities Press, 1965].

Winnicott, D. W. (1959–1964). La clasificación: ¿Hay una contribución psicoanalítica a la clasificación psiquiátrica? In: *Los procesos de maduración y el ambiente facilitador*. Buenos Aires: Paidós, 1993 [Classification: Is there a psychoanalytic contribution to psychiatric classification? In: *The Maturational Processes and the Facilitating Environment: Studies in the Theory of Emotional Development* (pp. 124–139). New York: International Universities Press, 1965].

Winnicott, D. W. (1960a). La teoría de la relación paterno filial. In: *Los procesos de maduración y el ambiente facilitador*. Buenos Aires: Paidós, 1993 [The theory of the parent-infant relationship. In: *The Maturational Processes and the Facilitating Environment: Studies in the Theory of Emotional Development* (pp. 37–55). New York: International Universities Press, 1965].

Winnicott, D. W. (1960b). La distorsión del yo en términos de self verdadero y falso. In: *Los procesos de maduración y el ambiente facilitador*. Buenos Aires: Paidós, 1993 [Ego distortion in terms of true and false self. In: *The Maturational Processes and the Facilitating Environment: Studies in the Theory of Emotional Development* (pp. 140–152). New York: International Universities Press, 1965].

Winnicott, D. W. (1960c). *La familia y el desarrollo del individuo*. Buenos Aires: Paidós, 1984 [*The Family and Individual Development*. London: Tavistock Publications, 1965].

Winnicott, D. W. (1961). Variedades de psicoterapia. In: *El hogar, nuestro punto de partida*. Buenos Aires: Paidós, 1993 [Varieties of psychotherapy. In: Winnicott, C., Shepherd, R., and Davis, M. (Eds.), *Deprivation and Delinquency* (pp. 232–240). London: Tavistock, 1984].

Winnicott, D. W. (1962). La integración del yo en el desarrollo del niño. In: Los procesos de maduración y el ambiente facilitador. Buenos Aires: Paidós, 1993 [Ego integration in child development. In: *The Maturational Processes and the Facilitating Environment: Studies in the Theory of Emotional Development* (pp. 56–63). New York: International Universities Press, 1965].

Winnicott, D. W. (1964). Importancia del encuadre en el modo de tratar la regresión en psicoanálisis. In: *Exploraciones Psicoanalíticas I*. Buenos Aires: Paidós, 1991

[The importance of the setting in meeting regression in psycho-analysis. In: Winnicott, C., Shepherd, R., and Davis, M. (Eds.), *Psycho-analytic Explorations* (pp. 96–102). Cambridge, MA: Harvard University Press, 1989].

Winnicott, D. W. (1964). *Exploraciones psicoanalíticas I*. Buenos Aires: Paidós, 1991 [*Psycho-analytic Explorations*. C. Winnicott, R. Shepherd, and M. Davis (Eds.). Cambridge, MA: Harvard University Press, 1989].

Winnicott, D. W. (1965a) El concepto de trauma en relación con el desarrollo del individuo dentro de la familia. In: *Exploraciones Psicoanalíticas I*. Buenos Aires: Paidós, 1991 [The concept of trauma in relation to the development of the individual within the family. In: Winnicott, C., Shepherd, R., and Davis, M. (Eds.), *Psycho-Analytic Explorations* (pp. 130–148). Cambridge, MA: Harvard University Press, 1989].

Winnicott, D. W. (1965b). Psicología de la locura. In: *Exploraciones Psicoanalíticas I*. Buenos Aires: Paidós, 1991 [The psychology of madness: A contribution from psychoanalysis. In: Winnicott, C., Shepherd, R., and Davis, M. (Eds.), *Psycho-Analytic Explorations* (pp. 119–129). Cambridge, MA: Harvard University Press, 1989].

Winnicott, D. W. (1965c). *The Family and Individual Development*. London: Tavistock.

Winnicott, D. W. (1966). Sobre los elementos masculino y femenino escindidos. Respuesta a comentarios. In: *Exploraciones Psicoanalíticas*. Buenos Aires: Paidós, 1991 [On split-off male and female elements to be found in men and women. In: Winnicott, C., Sheperd, R., and Davis, M. (Eds.), *Psychoanalytic Explorations* (pp. 169–188). Cambridge, MA: Harvard University Press, 1989].

Winnicott, D. W. (1967a). Posfacio: D.W.W. sobre D.W.W. In: *Exploraciones psicoanalíticas*. Buenos Aires: Paidós, 1991 [W.W. on D.W.W. In: C. Winnicott, R. Sheperd, and Davis, M. (Eds.), *Psychoanalytic Explorations* (pp. 569–583). Cambridge, MA: Harvard University Press, 1989].

Winnicott, D. W. (1967b). El concepto de individuo sano. In: *El hogar, nuestro punto de partida*. Buenos Aires: Paidós, 1993 [The concept of a healthy individual. In: Winnicott, C., Shepherd, R., and Davis, M. (Eds.), *Home Is Where We Start From: Essays by a Psychoanalyst* (pp. 21–34). New York and London: W. W. Norton, 1986].

Winnicott, D. W. (1970). Sobre las bases del Self en el cuerpo. In: *Exploraciones Psicoanalíticas I*. Buenos Aires: Paidós, 1991, pp. 322–323 [On the basis of self in body. In: Winnicott, C., Sheperd, R., and Davis, M. (Eds.), *Psychoanalytic Explorations* (pp. 261–271). Cambridge, MA: Harvard University Press, 1989].

Winnicott, D. W. (1971). *Playing and Reality*. London and New York: Routledge, 1989.

Winnicott, D. W. (1974). Fear of breakdown. *Int. Rev. Psycho-Anal.*, **1**: 103–107.

Winnicott, D. W. (1987). *Babies and Their Mothers*. Cambridge, MA: Perseus Publishing.

Winnicott, D. W. (1993). *Talking to Parents*. Winnicott, C. Bollas, C., Davis, M. and Shepherd, R. (Eds.), Reading, MA: Addison-Wesley, 1993.

Winograd, B. (2002). El psicoanálisis argentino [Argentine psychoanalysis]. Presented at the Fourth Argentine Psychoanalytic Conference], Rosario, May.

Winograd, B. (2005). *Depresión, ¿enfermedad o crisis?* [Depression – Illness or Crisis?]. Buenos Aires: Paidós.

Zak de Goldstein, R. (1996). El juego del señuelo, dimensión erótica del deseo [The game of the lure, erotic dimension of desire]. *Rev. de psicoanálisis.*, **53**(2): 493–503.

Zirlinger, S. (2001). Perturbaciones clínicas en la construcción de la realidad y la alteridad [Clinical disturbances in the construction of reality and alterity]. Retrieved from: www.winnicott.net.

Zirlinger, S. (2002). Una visión sintética sobre los aportes de D. Winnicott a la idea de la cura [A summarized view of D. W. Winnicott's contributions to the idea of the cure]. *Aperturas*, 12. Retrieved from: http://www.aperturas.org/autores. php?a=Zirlinger-Silvio.

Zukerfeld, R. (1988). Transferencia y sugestión [Transference and suggestion]. In: Braier, E. (Ed.), *Tabúes en teoría de la técnica* [Taboos in the Theory of Technique] (pp. 137–167). Buenos Aires: Nueva Visión, 1990.

Zukerfeld, R. (1999). Psicoanálisis actual: Tercera tópica, vulnerabilidad y contexto social [Current psychoanalysis: The third topography, vulnerability and social context]. *Aperturas*, 2. Retrieved from: http://www.aperturas.org/articulos. php?id=90&a=Psicoanalisis-actual-tercera-topica-vulnerabilidad-y-contexto-social.

Zukerfeld, R. (2002). Psicoanálisis, vulnerabilidad somática y resiliencia [Psychoanalysis, somatic vulnerability, and resiliency]. Presented at the Fourth Argentine Psychoanalytic Conference, Rosario, May.

Zukerfeld, R. and Zonis Zukerfeld, R. (1999). Procesos terciarios [Tertiary processes]. *Aperturas*, 14. Retrieved from http://www.aperturas.org/articulos.php?id=253&a=Procesos-terciarios

Zukerfeld, R. and Zonis Zukerfeld, R. (2004). Esperanza y determinismo en la actitud psicoanalítica: un estudio empírico sobre ciertos prejuicios teóricos [Hope and determinism in the psychoanalytic attitude: An empirical study on certain theoretical biases]. In: *Procesos Terciarios. De la vulnerabilidad a la resiliencia* [Tertiary Processes: From Vulnerability to Resiliency] (pp. 217–234). Buenos Aires: Lugar.

Appendix I
Major works by Winnicott

Clinical Notes on the Disorders of Childhood. London: Heinemann, 1931.

The Ordinary Devoted Mother and Her Baby: Nine Broadcast Talks (1949) (Private distribution only).

Collected Papers: Through Paediatrics to Psychoanalysis. London: Tavistock, 1957.

The Child and the Outside World: Studies in Developing Relationships. London: Tavistock, 1957.

On the contribution of direct child observation to psychoanalysis (1957). In: *The Maturational Processes and the Facilitating Environment: Studies in the Theory of Emotional Development* (pp. 109–114). New York: International Universities Press, 1965.

The Child and the Family: First Relationships. London: Tavistock, 1957.

The Child, the Family and the Outside World. Harmondsworth: Penguin, 1964.

The Maturational Processes and the Facilitating Environment: Studies in the Theory of Emotional Development. New York: International Universities Press, 1965.

The Family and Individual Development. London: Tavistock, 1965.

Playing and Reality. London: Tavistock, 1971.

Therapeutic Consultations in Child Psychiatry. London: Hogarth, 1971.

Fragment of an Analysis. New York: Grove Press, 1972.

The Piggle: An Account of the Psychoanalytic Treatment of a Little Girl. London: Hogarth and Madison, CT: International Universities Press, 1977.

Deprivation and Delinquency. London: Tavistock Publications, 1984.

Holding and Interpretation. London: Hogarth and the Inst. of PSA, 1986; New York: Grove Press, 1987; reprinted London: The Inst. of PSA and Karnac Books, 1989.

Home is Where We Start from: Essays by a Psychoanalyst, Winnicott, C., Shepherd, R., & Davis, M. (Eds). New York & London: W.W. Norton; Harmondsworth: Penguin, 1986.

Babies and their Mothers, Winnicott, C., Shepherd, R., & Davis, M. (Eds). Reading, MA: Addison-Wesley, 1987.

The Spontaneous Gesture, Selected Letters. Rodman, F. R. (Ed.). London & Cambridge, MA: Harvard University Press, 1987.

Human Nature. London: Free Association Books; New York: Schocken Books, 1988; reprinted New York: Brunner/Mazel, 1991.

Psychoanalytic Explorations. London: Karnac Books; Cambridge, MA: Harvard University Press, 1989.

Talking to Parents. Winnicott, C. Bollas, C., Davis, M. and Shepherd, R. (Eds.), Reading, MA: Addison-Wesley, 1993.

Thinking about Children. Shepherd, R., Johns, J., & Taylor Robinson, H. (Eds.), London: Karnac Books, 1996.

Appendix II

Relevant works by Kohut and further reading on Kohut's ideas

Works by Kohut

Kohut, H. and Levarie, S. (1950). On the enjoyment of listening to music. *Psychoanal. Q.*, **19**: 64–87.

Kohut, H. (1952). Book review of *Psychanalyse de la Musique. Psychoanal. Q.*, **21**: 109–111.

Kohut, H. (1955). Book review of *Beethoven and His Nephew., Psychoanal. Q.*, **24**: 453–455.

Kohut, H. (1955). Book review of *The Haunting Melody. Psychoanalytic Experiences in Life and Music. Psychoanal. Q.*, **24**: 134–137.

Kohut, H. (1957). *Death in Venice* by Mann: Disintegration of artistic sublimation. *Psychoanal. Q.*, **26**: 206–228.

Kohut, H. (1957). Observations on the psychological functions of music. *J. Amer. Psychoanal. Assn.*, **5**: 389–407.

Kohut, H. (1957). Panel report: Clinical and theoretical aspects of resistance. *J. Amer. Psychoanal. Assn.*, **5**: 548–555.

Kohut, H. (1957). Book review of *The Arrow and the Lyre. A Study of the Role of Love in the Works of Thomas Mann. Psychoanal. Q.*, **26**: 273–275.

Kohut, H. (1959). Introspection, empathy, and psychoanalysis. *J. Amer. Psychoanal. Assn.*, **7**: 459–483.

Kohut, H. (1960). Book review of *Beethoven and his Nephew: A Psychoanalytic Study of their Relationship. J. Amer. Psychoanal. Assn.*, **8**: 567–586.

Kohut, H. (1960). Panel report: The psychology of imagination. *J. Amer. Psychoanal. Assn.*, **8**: 159–166.

Kohut, H. (1962). The psychoanalytic curriculum. *J. Amer. Psychoanal. Assn.*, **10**: 153–163.

Kohut, H. (1964). Phyllis Greenacre - a tribute. *J. Amer. Psychoanal. Assn.*, **12**: 3–5.

Kohut, H. (1964). Symposium on fantasy. *Int. J. Psychoanal.*, **45**: 199–202.

Kohut, H. (1966). Forms and transformations of narcissism. *J. Amer. Psychoanal. Assn.*, **14**: 243–272.

Kohut, H. (1968). Narcissistic personality disorders: Outline of a systematic approach. *Psychoanal. Study Child*, **23**: 86–113.

Kohut, H. (1968). The evaluation of applicants for psychoanalytic training. *Int. J. Psychoanal.*, **49**: 548–554.

Kohut, H. (1970). Scientific activities of the American psychoanalytic association. *J. Amer. Psychoanal. Assn.*, **18**: 462–484.

Kohut, H. (1971a). Peace prize 1969: Laudation. *J. Amer. Psychoanal. Assn.*, **19**: 806–818.

Kohut, H. (1971b). *The Analysis of the Self. A Systematic Approach to the Psychoanalytic Treatment of Narcissistic Personality Disorders.* New York: International Universities Press.

Kohut, H. (1972). Thoughts on narcissism and narcissistic rage. *Psychoanal. Study Child*, **27**: 360–400.

Kohut, H. (1973). Psychoanalysis in a troubled world. *Ann. Psychoanal.*, **1**: 3–25.

Kohut, H. (1975). The future of psychoanalysis. *Ann. Psychoanal.*, **3**: 325–340.

Kohut, H. (1975). The psychoanalyst in the community of scholars. *Ann. Psychoanal.*, **3**: 341–370.

Kohut, H. (1976). Creativeness, charisma, group psychology: Freud's self-analysis. *Psychol. Issues*, **34**: 379–425.

Kohut, H. (1977). On the occasion of Jean Piaget's eightieth birthday. *Ann. Psychoanal.*, **5**: 373–378.

Kohut, H. (1977). *The Restoration of the Self.* New York: International Universities Press.

Kohut, H. and Wolf, E. S. (1978). The disorders of the self and their treatment: An outline. *Int. J. Psychoanal.*, **59**: 413–426.

Kohut, H. (1978). *The Search for the Self: Selected Writings of Heinz Kohut, 1950–1978, 2 Vols.* Ornstein, P. (Ed.), New York: International Universities Press.

Kohut, H. (1979). The two analysis of Mr. Z. *Int. J. Psychoanal.*, **60**: 3–27.

Kohut, H. (1982). Introspection, empathy and the semi-circle of mental health. *Int. J. Psychoanal.*, **63**: 395–407.

Kohut, H. (1984). *How Does Analysis Cure?* Goldberg, A. (Ed.), Chicago & London: University of Chicago Press.

Kohut, H. (1985). *Self Psychology and the Humanities: Reflections on a New Psychoanalytic Approach.* Strozier, C. (Ed.), New York & London: W. W. Norton.

Kohut, H. (ed. P. Ornstein) (1991). *The Search for the Self: Selected Writings of Heinz Kohut, 4 Vols.* New York: International Universities Press.

Cocks, G. (Ed.) (1994). *The Curve of Life: Correspondence of Heinz Kohut, 1923–1981.* Chicago: University of Chicago Press.

Further Reading on Kohut

Adler, G. (1989). Uses and limitations of Kohut's self psychology in the treatment of borderline patients. *J. Amer. Psychoanal. Assn.*, **37**: 761–786.

Bacal, H. A. (1995). The essence of Kohut's work and the progress of self psychology. *Psychoanal. Dialogues*, **5**: 353–366.

Basch, M. F. (1984). Memorial for Heinz Kohut, M.D., October 31, 1981. *Ann. Psychoanal.*, **12**: 5–8.

Basch, M. F. (1995). Kohut's contribution. *Psychoanal. Dialogues*, **5**: 367–374.

Baudry, F. (1998). Kohut and Glover: The role of subjectivity in psychoanalytic theory and controversy. *Psychoanal. Study Child*, **53**: 3–24.

Chessick, R. D. (1980). The problematical self in Kant and Kohut. *Psychoanal. Q.*, **49**: 456–473.

Chessick, R. D. (1988). A comparison of the notion of self in the philosophy of Heidegger and the psychoanalytic self psychology of Kohut. *Psychoanal. Contemp. Thought*, **11**: 117–144.

Ehrlich, R. (1985). Social dimensions of Heinz Kohut's psychology of the self. *Psychoanal. Contemp. Thought*, **8**: 333–354.

Elson, M. (Ed.) (1987). *The Kohut Seminars on Self Psychology and Psychotherapy with Adolescents and Young Adults*. New York: W. W. Norton.

Friedman, L. (1986). Kohut's testament. *Psychoanal. Inquiry*, **6**: 321–348.

Gagnier, T. T. and Robertiello, R. C. (1983). Klein and Kohut: Clinical confluence-theoretical differences. *Psychoanal. Rev.*, **70**: 372–386.

Gedo, J. E. (1975). To Heinz Kohut: On his 60th birthday. *Ann. Psychoanal.*, **3**: 313–324.

Glassman, M. (1988). Kernberg and Kohut: Competing psychoanalytic models of narcissism. *J. Amer. Psychoanal. Assn.*, **36**: 597–626.

Goldberg, A. (Ed.) (1978). *The Psychology of the Self: A Casebook. Written with the Collaboration of Heinz Kohut*. New York: International Universities Press.

Goldberg, A. (Ed.) (1983). *The Future of Psychoanalysis: Essays in Honor of Heinz Kohut*. New York: International Universities Press.

Goldberg, A. (Ed.) (1988). *Learning from Kohut*. Hillsdale, NJ: The Analytic Press.

Goldberg, A. (1998). Self psychology since Kohut. *Psychoanal. Q.*, **67**: 240–255.

Hamburg, P. (1991). Interpretation and empathy: Reading Lacan and Kohut. *Int. J. Psychoanal.*, **72**: 347–362.

Jacoby, M. (1990). *Individuation and Narcissism: The Psychology of the Self in Jung and Kohut*. London: Routledge.

Kirsner, D. (1982). Self psychology and psychoanalysis: Interview with Heinz Kohut. *Psychoanal. Contemp. Thought*, **5**: 483–495.

Kligerman, C. (1984). Heinz Kohut: A dedication. *Ann. Psychoanal.*, **12**: 3–4.

Kligerman, C. (1984). Memorial for Heinz Kohut, M. D., October 31, 1981. *Ann. Psychoanal.*, **12**: 9–18.

Kramer, S. and Akhtar, S. (1994). *Mahler and Kohut: Perspectives on Development, Psychopathology, and Technique*. Northvale, NJ: Jason Aronson.

Lee, R. R. and Martin, J. C. (1991). *Psychotherapy after Kohut: A Textbook of Self Psychology*. Hillsdale, NJ: The Analytic Press.

Modell, A. (1986). The missing element in Kohut's cure. *Psychoanal. Inquiry*, **6**: 367–386.

Munschauer, C. A. (1987). A bridge between the theories of Kernberg and Kohut. *Psychoanal. Inquiry*, **7**: 99–120.

Ornstein, P. H. (1974). Narcissistic personality disorders: Kohut's contribution. *Ann. Psychoanal.*, **2**: 127–149.

Ornstein, P. H. and Ornstein, A. (1995). Some distinguishing features of Heinz Kohut's self psychology. *Psychoanal. Dialogues*, **5**: 385–392.

Saperstein, J. and Gaines, J. (1978). Commentary on divergent views of Kernberg and Kohut. *Int. Rev. Psychoanal.*, **5**: 413–424.

Siegel, A. (1996). *Heinz Kohut and the Psychology of the Self*. London & New York: Routledge.

Simpson, P. (1994). Heinz Kohut: His enduring influence today. *Psychoanal. Psychother. Rev.*, **5**(1): 6–23.

Stepansky, P. E. (1983). Dissent: Adler, Kohut and psychoanalytic research tradition. *Ann. Psychoanal.*, **11**: 51–76.

Stepansky, P. and Goldberg, A. (Eds.) (1984). *Kohut's Legacy. Contributions to Self Psychology.* Hillsdale, NJ: The Analytic Press.

Tonkin, M. and Fine, H. J. (1985). Narcissism and borderline states: Kernberg, Kohut, psychotherapy. *Psychoanal. Psychol.*, **2**: 221–240.

Treurniet, N. (1980). Concepts of self and ego in Kohut's psychology of the self. *Int. J. Psychoanal.*, **61**: 325–334.

Index

Note: Page numbers followed by "n" denote endnotes.

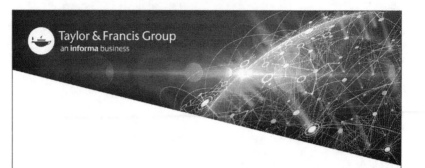

Taylor & Francis Group
an **informa** business

Taylor & Francis eBooks

www.taylorfrancis.com

A single destination for eBooks from Taylor & Francis
with increased functionality and an improved user
experience to meet the needs of our customers.

90,000+ eBooks of award-winning academic content in
Humanities, Social Science, Science, Technology, Engineering,
and Medical written by a global network of editors and authors.

TAYLOR & FRANCIS EBOOKS OFFERS:

A streamlined
experience for
our library
customers

A single point
of discovery
for all of our
eBook content

Improved
search and
discovery of
content at both
book and
chapter level

REQUEST A FREE TRIAL
support@taylorfrancis.com

 Routledge
Taylor & Francis Group

 CRC Press
Taylor & Francis Group